INSTINCTIVE FITNESS

A re-evolutionary approach to **AGELESS HEALTH** and **FITNESS** based on a 2.5 million year experiment

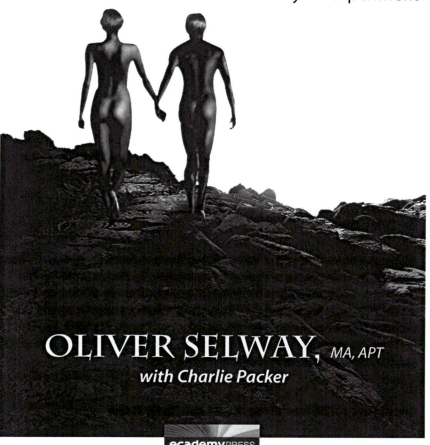

OLIVER SELWAY, MA, APT

with Charlie Packer

ecademyPRESS
www.ecademy-press.com

INSTINCTIVE FITNESS
A re-evolutionary approach to **AGELESS HEALTH** and **FITNESS**
based on a 2.5 million year experiment

First published in 2012 by
Ecademy Press
48 St Vincent Drive, St Albans, Herts, AL1 5SJ
info@ecademy-press.com
www.ecademy-press.com

Printed and bound by Lightning Source in the UK and USA
Cover Illustration and design by Michael Inns/Oliver Selway
Artwork by Karen Gladwell

Printed on acid-free paper from managed forests.

ISBN 978-1-9078746-04-7

INSTINCTIVE FITNESS

A re-evolutionary approach to **AGELESS HEALTH** and **FITNESS**
based on a 2.5 million year experiment

Dedication

This book is dedicated to my parents to whom I have been even more of a burden as an adult than as a child. Without their support, there would be no me, no book and no point.

Contents

Disclaimer

The lawyers want me to say…

The information provided in this book should not be construed as personal medical advice or instruction. No action should be taken based solely on the contents of this book.

Readers should consult appropriate health professionals on any matter relating to their health and well-being.

The information and opinions provided here are believed to be accurate and sound and are based on the best judgments of the authors, but readers who fail to consult appropriate health authorities assume the risk of any injuries.
The author does not accept liability for errors or omissions.

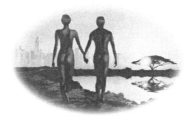

Acknowledgements

This isn't meant to an anatomy book or a biochemistry primer, instead it is an introduction to what I consider to be the most powerful approach to Fitness and Health *anybody* can take. In essence it's a book of observations and ideas, and as such it contains some oversimplifications in places; I hope more 'sciencey' readers will forgive me for these.

I wanted this book to be for the man or woman in the street, giving them the motivation to just to get going, without getting bogged down in trying to understand the minutiae of the chemical reactions that occur in the body or having to choose between hundreds of different exercise routines.

Just as anyone can get on an aeroplane and benefit from the power of flight without having to understand aeronautical physics or how the cockpit works, I haven't written a pilot's instructional course, but rather, I hope, a good guide for passengers contemplating their first flight.

Having said that, if you follow the references provided you can look even deeper into the weight of scientific evidence that underpins the Instinctive Fitness approach – even if few people are yet making practical use of it.

This book does not appear in a vacuum, and I am deeply indebted to the work of a number of writers and bloggers who have inspired me and have done much to popularise the Paleo movement – a revolutionary new way of thinking that has made serious inroads in the US and is now gradually spreading across to the UK. (As usual, we are a few years behind on this side of the pond.)

In this category lies the genius **Mark Sisson** in California, who blogs harder for the Paleo community than anyone on the planet. He promotes what he calls a 'Primal' approach, but we share the same emphasis on looking at our evolutionary past and designing lifestyles that take this golden age in our history as their cue.

I hope he comes across this book and that it meets with his approval. He is an inspiration.

Another figure who has helped re-launch the 'caveman' lifestyle is **Erwan Le Corre**, a Frenchman living in the USA. His emphasis on moving naturally in the natural environment represents the furthest and most radical application of the logic I employ in this book.

Authors **Robb Wolf** and **Loren Cordain** are the leading lights of the Paleo dietary movement in the US and have done much to bring approaches similar to those outlined in this book into the lives of their fellow countrymen.

I used to be a fan of the Alexander Technique but I found it to be too difficult and time consuming. I now believe that the future of non-surgical spinal care and the search for natural human posture lies with the work of **Esther Gokhale**. I have used some of her ideas in my description of what people can do to escape the clutches of back pain and arthritis, and to improve their general athletic performance.

To all of the above, I often feel like I am standing on the shoulders of giants; your influence changed the way I think about the human body forever. For that I thank you.

Lastly, closer to home, I want to thank **Charlie Packer** for taking my bag of ideas and helping me turn them into both a book and whole movement. His tireless help with massaging my dry prose into something that catches the readers' imagination has brought out the full potential of the Instinctive Fitness vision. All his efforts and talents are much in evidence here.

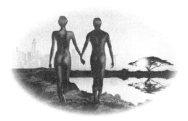

Introduction

Despite a multi-billion pound health and fitness industry and all the wonders of modern health care, modern day humans rank as the weakest, flabbiest, most disease-prone and stressed-out animal ever to walk the earth.

Yet this lamentable decline in society's physical wellbeing during the 21st century is an entirely preventable tragedy that could easily be reversed.

It's clear to me that the modern commercial world is leading our natural animal instincts astray – tempting us, teasing us, ensnaring us and ultimately betraying us with empty promises. Our hard-wired animal instincts unconsciously control so much of our behaviour, but only by understanding the nature of the modern world we live in can they be made to work for, rather than against us.

I'm going to explain how the establishment's attempts to micro-manage our eating habits have contributed far more harm than good, damaging our innate sense of what's right for us. The scandalous truth is that ageing, obesity and the vast majority of modern health ailments are due to neither lack of effort nor the passing of years but to the fact we've all been brainwashed into believing things that, as Mark Twain wrote, 'just ain't so'.

Endless cardio, low-fat diets, hours of working out and boring cuisine are unnecessary, burdensome or even downright dangerous. In fact, high levels of fitness and health aren't something we must stress, strive and invariably pay hard cash for. They are available to all of us when we start choosing the right kinds of food and doing the right kinds of exercise.

No matter what your age or gender, a personal transformation is possible. We can, with the application of a little thought, reason and self-awareness, re-harness our basic human drives to unleash once again the physical grandeur that is our birth right.

Looking back at evolutionary history, there's clear evidence that ancient humans were physically superior to those we know today. They were healthy, vibrant and powerful beings from whom we should learn how to restore the physical splendour nature intended us to enjoy.

We live in a modern world radically different to that of our ancient ancestors – but our unchanged Stone Age genes yearn for the same challenges and environment they faced. The lifestyle of our modern world is detrimental to our health in many ways; however, there is an answer if we look back and learn from the past...

The personal discovery that transformed my own life was that health, energy and body composition can quickly be restored to the way nature intended simply by choosing a healthy, high-fat, medium protein, low carb diet and relying mainly on easy, relaxing exercise; in other words, treating our bodies in the way in which they are evolutionarily best adapted.

With just a subtle change of attitude and a proper understanding of how your body works best, you can free yourself from commercial and nutritional exploitation and transform yourself from the inside out.

*This ancient, time-tested approach will help you regain control of the **animal instincts** that served your ancestors so well for thousands of years - eating like a king, playing like a child and living your life to the full!*

Instinctive Fitness is not another rigid prescription for health
and fitness, and I'm no self-proclaimed expert
(of which we have quite enough already).

*"Trust your own instinct. Your mistakes might as well
be your own, instead of someone else's."*

Billy Wilder

CHAPTER ONE

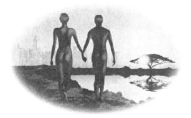

Basic Instinct!

*"Nothing in biology makes sense,
except in the light of evolution"*

Theodosius Dobzhandsky
(geneticist and evolutionary biologist)

Once upon a time, not so long ago, a not-quite-as-young-as-he-used-to-be man stepped out of his morning shower, wrapped a towel around his waist and strode confidently into the bedroom to get dressed, just as he'd always done. Nonchalantly glancing across the room, he caught a reflection in his full length mirror that knocked him for six! Lurking where the trim, fit and athletic man once stood was an unfamiliar imposter who appeared to be none of those things.

The not-so-young man grudgingly lowered his eyes to fully take in the imposter's flabby girth, and gave his man boobs a little wobble just to confirm they weren't the relaxed muscle he'd hoped they were. He thought to himself, "I wasn't like this yesterday – was I?" This was truly shocking! How could all his frantic efforts in the gym to maintain his youthful shape be failing so badly? And why had he not noticed this before? With the weight of a dumbbell he so often worked out with in the gym, a thought slammed into his head: "If I'm like this now, what on earth will I be like when I'm sixty?!"

Never having craved the appearance of a professional bodybuilder, bulging biceps were not something he'd ever strived for, yet what stood before him was preposterous; he couldn't even recognise this skinny-fat body. (You know the look - skinny arms and shoulders accompanied by a spreading midriff).

Deep down he'd known his energy levels were no longer what they had been when he was a competitive athlete in his teens, but this overpowering feeling of deflation was something completely new. It suddenly dawned on him that even with regular exercise and a 'sensible' diet, the best years of his life were quite obviously now far behind.

However, this deflated feeling didn't last long, and his disappointment and embarrassment quickly turned into feeling of having being ripped off and short changed. Frankly, he was furious; not because he had brought this on by inactivity, eating junk food and letting himself get horribly overweight (this isn't one of those stories), but because he *was* active and he *was* eating what he'd been lead to believe were the right things!

The hours of training he was putting in each week were obviously no longer cutting it, and were seemingly making little headway into fending off those now nicely developing little love handles. What was going on? He was running lots, regularly knocking out press-ups and squats while fastidiously avoiding saturated fat – all the things the 'experts' were telling him were the keys to fitness and health!

All his life he had carefully followed these 'golden rules' and the accepted wisdom that pours out from the government and media: wisdom he had once thought was the very reason he *had* always been so trim, but now it was seemingly getting him nowhere!

"This must be the way of things," he concluded. "Despite our best efforts, we're all doomed to that middle aged spread". And as a wave of stoic defeatism rolled over him, for a moment he contemplated welcoming in this inevitable decline into middle-age stodginess with an extra couple of Weetabix for breakfast.

But then something snapped in his head!

He said to himself, "There must be another way to go about this; there has to be something fundamentally wrong with what we're all being told. There must be a way of getting into and maintaining a great shape without all the effort, pain and anguish."

That man – as you might have guessed – was me.

Only two months later, without committing any extra time or effort to training, I was a different man. I had found my own Holy Grail: a way to lose fat and gain muscle *at the same time*. There was almost no supporting evidence in the mainstream media to back up the methods I used, but it was clear that my newly formulated dietary and exercise methods had resulted in the loss of all the fat I had accumulated over the last decade in just a few weeks, whilst developing new muscle that people quickly started noticing.

The pictures below aren't truly representative, as I didn't pre-plan this transformation, but they do give an idea of how I once again became proud of my own body.

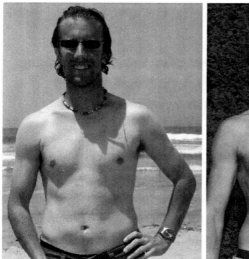 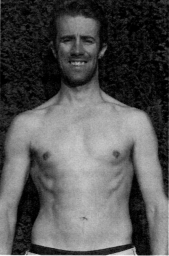

Sure, I don't look like Stallone (I don't think I want to either), but this new, fitter leaner me was about *much* more than just looks. The benefits extended to *amazing* athletic performance: at 34 I was fitter than I had ever been, and fitter than anyone else I knew. I was even stronger, faster and more athletic than I had been at sixteen when I was the 1500m Bucks County Athletics Champion.

This isn't fanciful thinking – I proved it. To test myself, I entered the *same* county athletics event *18 years after I had last competed in it* and ran 4 minutes 32 seconds – bettering my old personal best by a small margin. This was done after only 8 weeks' of my newly adopted methods of eating and training.

I now had an abundance of energy and well-being that I hadn't experienced in decades; the layer of fat I'd been steadily collecting around my midriff had, as if by magic, disappeared. I started feeling 'right' in myself again and my lost confidence quickly returned. My body started feeling like mine again, rather than that awkward, strangely-shaped vehicle I'd grudgingly begun accepting as mine.

> *Ok, so you got yourself into great shape*, you might be thinking that's kind of impressive but o*thers have done so before – so what?*

Yes, but here's the rub:

> *I achieved all this without effort, extra hours training,*
> *low-calorie dieting, boring meal choices or*
> *fancy (and expensive) gym membership.*

Moreover, 3 years on and aged almost 37, I have *maintained* this shape and fitness level almost effortlessly, whilst everybody else I have seen make improvements during this time have slipped back into their previous habits and returned to their previous low levels of fitness within a matter of months. It turns out that the method I stumbled upon, as well as delivering consistent results, has an added quality that changes everything. I call it *stickability*: a quality that separates winners from losers in all endeavours.

I found out that when you make the *right changes*, you'll be able to keep all the progress you make. Get there the wrong way and all you'll get is a temporary fix before your body and your habits snap back to where you started like an elastic band.

I was so excited by my discovery that I quit my job in journalism there and then to qualify and share my knowledge as a Personal Trainer. I was desperate to pass this knowledge on to as many people as I could, and I was over the moon when my methods worked equally well for *everyone* I worked with; from young, active sportsmen and women, right through to older members of society who were starting from a much lower base level of fitness the results were always the same: huge gains in health, fitness and vitality in an astonishingly short time.

Are you curious to know how this happened?

Let me explain what I did:

Sick of being 'skinny-fat' - I decided to 'sort matters out'; however, I couldn't decide what training system to use. I mean there are thousands of different opinions on the right way to go, and none of them sounded right to me. I wanted something that actually worked, and being a researcher, I naturally read thousands of articles and checked out hundreds of websites, getting more and more confused until I finally stumbled onto a truth that rocked me to my core.

It was a truth that took some digging out because it wasn't widely publicised, and it wasn't making national headlines – not because it didn't work, but because it didn't involve selling anything: no dietary supplements, no special exercise machines and no television series! Like a lot of great ideas, it was lost because…

…it was never going to make anyone any money!

The penny only dropped when I started to ask the one question that no-one seems to ask - *why* **is it necessary for humans to make an effort to get fit at all**? After all, it's not like wild animals have an exercise programme:

> *I've never seen an Iguana going hard-core with weights*
> *or a Snow Leopard warming up before heading out*
> *for a 'light jog'.*

It was *then* that I had my Eureka moment. I realised that no other animal on this planet stresses about its fitness: they don't count the calories, worry about nutrition or ask if their hips look too big! No, they simply do what they do, and remain at peak fitness by doing what they have evolved to do: living active lives, eating all the nutritious food they crave and leaving plenty of time for rest and play.

I concluded that the real issue is that modern people no longer live the lives they evolved to lead and that many of the instincts that we relied on for millennia are now missing the environment that made them useful. Many of our drives are now therefore misaligned with the behaviour they evolved to produce. These ancient instincts now drive us to develop modern habits of eating, moving and living for which they were never intended.

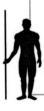

Our modern world is thousands of years more advanced than our bodies which are unchanged since the Paleolithic times; while we're sitting on the sofa scoffing sandwiches, our Stone Age body is expecting us to be out hunting and foraging, resting and playing – the only sorts of exercise we needed to take for hundreds of thousands of years.

With this insight, everything suddenly became clear to me: in order to live up to our highest potential as humans and members of the animal kingdom, we need to look to the past – not to technology – to get fit.

I'm suggesting that we shouldn't be vainly searching for something 'new' to fight heart disease, obesity and diabetes, and instead we should simply look back into our past and re-discover what made our ancient ancestors supremely fit, healthy and disease free![1]

Evolution confusion

We humans got to where we are today not through thinking or inventing our way to the top, but through the multimillion year process of evolution. However, we should not mistake this for any 'grand plan' of conscious design, but we should consider it instead as a very long series of minor anomalies which, when multiplied and compounded over millions of years, created enormous variations in the species of animals.

When placed into the context of an animal's specific environment, these seemingly minor adaptations caused the animal to have either a statistically better or worse chance of flourishing and passing on that characteristic on to the next generation.

Over the millennia these minor changes resulted in a steady divergence of physical characteristics between two groups of animals, until what once would have been considered the very same animal had become a completely separate species. And so it was with Homo Sapiens.

These evolutionary changes are not restricted just to *physical* adaptations visible to the naked eye; they also include *behaviour*. A genetic quirk might furnish a species with more aggressive hunting skills, better adaptations to nurture their young, a taste for a new type of food, or a better defence against a predatory species – anything that increases their chances of living long enough to produce the next generation.

Each species of animal on this planet has its own hard-wired set of rules they must obey: bats wake up at dusk, spiders spin webs and bears hibernate during winter. They don't think about what they are doing – these are simply the rules they must follow no matter what.

However, any of these behaviours, when removed from the correct context of their natural habitat, can lead the creature astray: a turkey obediently nurturing a wooden egg, a magpie risking everything to collect shiny man-made objects, or a domesticated dog compelled to turn round and round to flatten non-existent grass before settling down in its blanket-covered bed.

> Each behavioural pattern has a very good reason in the wild – but let loose in an alien environment it can become counterproductive or even self-harming.

And so it is for humans

Our own human instincts have, since the agricultural and industrial revolutions, been denied their natural environment. This leaves us with certain impulses and deep-seated desires that no longer serve us in this new, complicated, commercially-driven world.

Although we consider ourselves superior to any other species with our ability to *reason* out our actions, on closer inspection, man is not so very different to other animals. Under a thin layer of conscious thought lie the same hard-wired animal responses which so often dictate the *real* reasons for our behaviour. This leaves our so-called intelligent, conscious mind the unenviable task of rationalising our actions *after* they've been played out.

Primitive behavioural drivers

It's all very well referring to 'instincts' and behaviours - but what actually *drives* animals to act in the way they do? It seems to me that all behaviours, whether animal or human, are driven by very simple risk/reward, carrot/ stick motivations: we do what makes us feel most comfortable at the time. Pavlov proved many years ago in his experiments with dogs that they can be conditioned to salivate in reaction to a meaningless bell-ringing stimulus when it is linked in the dog's mind to a reward. I believe that the physical body has its own specific tricks, signals and incentives to elicit the brain to respond with the actions it requires – and each of the signals the body sends out ultimately has both stick and carrot forms. Here are some basic examples:

Hunger

Stick: Hunger pains, irritability, low energy

Carrot: The good taste of food and the satisfaction of feeling full

Sleep

Stick: Lethargy, achiness, irritability and all the other symptoms of tiredness

Carrot: The warm, cosy feeling you get when drifting off to sleep.

Hunt

Stick: Associations with hunger feelings, itchy feet to chase prey.

Carrot: The endorphins released during the 'high' of the hunt, the thrill of the kill and the satisfaction of eating and sharing with the family and tribe.

Sex

I'm sure I don't need to explain this one, but you get the idea!

You see at a very fundamental level, I believe the body itself knows what it needs at any given time and provides a push to the mind to carry out the actions it thinks are in its own best interests. During the Stone Age, when our instincts were tuned to perfection, this all worked extremely well, but...

Unfortunately in this very confusing modern world the well-meaning carrot and stick instructions the body dishes out are no longer serving us quite as intended.

Our instincts balanced to our environment.

For millions of years our natural environment subjected us to specific challenges, and to survive our instincts and behaviours grew attuned to meet these challenges by the hard-nosed 'live or die' rules of evolution. We are in essence like any other creatures – reacting impulsively and without thinking when faced with certain circumstances. Many thousands of years ago these impulsive, instinctual actions were undoubtedly the right ones for our *natural* environment.

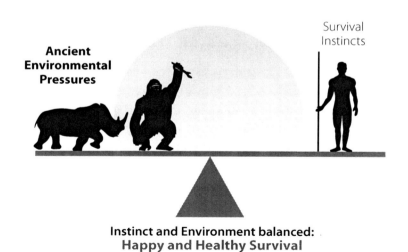

Ancient Environmental Pressures

Survival Instincts

Instinct and Environment balanced:
Happy and Healthy Survival

Our incompatible world: *Instinct versus modern living*

However the modern world has grown to confuse and corrupt our deepest human instincts. We like to think of ourselves as existing on a higher plane to our animal cousins, but underneath all the trinkets of modern living, in an older, deeper part of the brain, we are still the same animal we always were, running on the exact same programming.

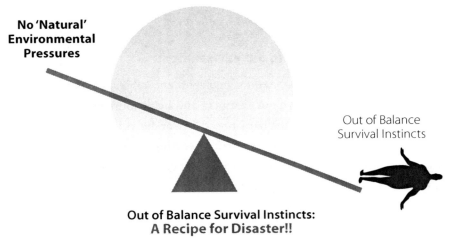

No 'Natural' Environmental Pressures

Out of Balance Survival Instincts

Out of Balance Survival Instincts: A Recipe for Disaster!!

The same instincts that kept us alive in ancient times are now being deliberately played by a modern world they simply weren't designed for.

Are we really so unlike the animals?

It's so easy to see that particular animals have certain built-in responses that cause them to act predictably in a variety of circumstances. Salmon will swim upstream to spawn at a precise time of the year; most animals will fight anything that threatens their offspring; a cornered animal will fight, run, or play dead; and most animals have built-in food-seeking behaviour and complex but identical courtship rituals for mating. It's almost like they are acting out a script written hundreds of thousands of years ago.

A cuckoo chick is a good example. Implanted into another bird's nest by its mother, it will always seek to push rival chicks out of the nest to their death. It's in their genes. Nobody blames these animals for any of these actions - they are just playing out the instincts that nature built into them.

Humans, however – or so the theories go – can exercise reason, awareness and conscious control over their behaviours. Indeed, our whole system of law is built on the idea that we can be held accountable for our actions. But all too often we find ourselves acting against our best interests and the idea that we are masters of our souls, captains of our destiny and the architects of our own lives quickly starts to slip. We find ourselves taking actions that can only be explained by saying "I felt like it" no matter how little sense the action makes from an objective, long-term, self-interested perspective.

We feel the shame of making the wrong decision, but we do it anyway, controlled by inner forces greater than our conscious, rationalising mind.

These sorts of actions, driven by basic human urges that we once depended on for survival, now cause a host of modern problems. These instincts, once finely balanced against the harsh reality of surviving an ancient world, now inadvertently wreak havoc in our everyday lives.

The sorts of challenges we once faced, and that evolution prepared us for, no longer exist for us. Instead, these basic drives have been hijacked by technology and commerce, actually damaging us rather than helping us to thrive:-

> To find true health in the modern world we need to understand the nature of our innate human instincts forged in a Stone Age environment. We need to find ways to realign those drives with the stimulation, challenges and nutrition that our bodies evolved to thrive on.
>
> We also need to immunise ourselves from the modern threats, lures, baits and traps waiting to hook us into the false comforts of modern living.

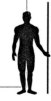

The ancient drives that served us well for millions of years are not always obvious, as they've been bent out of shape and abused by modern living, but they do exist, and by becoming aware of them, you will start to respect them more, understand what they are trying to do for you, and look for ways to defend them against exploitation.

Ten Basic Human Survival Instincts

Rest whenever possible

Eat whatever's available and tastes good

*Put on weight whenever possible
in case of famine*

*Crave sweet things because they contain
essential vitamins*

*Crave salty things because we need
the minerals*

Crave fatty foods for energy

Consume whatever looks bright and healthy

Go to sleep when it's dark

Wake up when it's light

*Copy the postures and movement
of those around us*

Because of the way technology and commerce has changed our modern world beyond the scope of these hard-wired urges, our instincts are constantly being tricked and so lead us badly astray. We are left open to deliberate exploitation by the food industry, the drug industry, advertising, baseless nutritional theories and other forces that only have their own interests at heart. Here's where each of these instincts get hijacked.

Our Instincts - *Hijacked, Corrupted and Misaligned*

Rest whenever possible: The world we live in today offers us few of the physical challenges of the natural environment, so we are no longer forced to raise our physical game. Our jobs, daily chores and even our leisure activities offer up little requirement to flex our muscles and tax our bodies in any way – leaving our inherent desire to rest and relax whenever possible woefully out of balance with the necessities of survival.

Eat whatever is available and tastes good: All modern food is designed to titillate the palate in a way that over-stimulates the brain's pleasure receptors. The chemical reactions elicited in the brain set up a chemical dependency and a psychological addiction that are as difficult for some to forsake as hard drugs. This sort of food is now available 24/7 from any supermarket. In the past, the changing seasons which once brought many exciting textures and flavours to our palate served to ensure that we always benefited from a varying nutritional profile through the year. Today, we restrict our diet to those foods we like best and we're able to obtain our favourite 'poisons' all year round.

Put on weight whenever possible: Our ancient relatives' craving for calories was essential for their survival because they could never be sure when the next meal was coming along. Today – secure in the knowledge that the next meal is probably already in the fridge, the cupboard or perhaps even on its way to being delivered hot to the front door – this binge-balancing famine never comes.

Crave sweet foods: One of nature's ways of telling us something is fit for consumption is by making it sweet. This instinct encouraged us to eat fruit and honey when it was available, along with any sweet tasting meat. (Many meats do taste sweet if your mind hasn't been conditioned to compare them to sugary bags of Haribo!) Today, nearly all packaged food tastes tantalisingly sweet because it's artificially enhanced with added sugars and sweeteners (not to mention the other MSGs and other carefully-selected addictive substances the food industry has knowingly adopted.)

Crave salty foods: Our drive to consume food with a salty taste would have led us to consume salty meats, sea salt or shellfish – all highly beneficial foods. Our love of this taste may have evolved to guard against a lack of minerals, such as sodium, magnesium, calcium or potassium, in our diet. Nowadays, however, it drives us to consume any sort of processed garbage that's been covered in cheap salt, stripped of any naturally available minerals in the manufacturing process. Of course, no amount of fake salt will ever supply us with the minerals found in real salt, or the essential vitamins and minerals found in the meats that contain this taste, so our drive for salty foods gets stuck in an endless, addictive loop.

Crave Fatty Foods: Our desire to consume fatty foods makes perfect evolutionary sense. We evolved to use this as our main fuel when we were big game hunters on the African savannah. However, many products today contain fat mixed with sugar in a way that nature never provides. Ice-cream, for example, gives us the fat we crave while simultaneously filling us with addictively high levels of sugar that damage our palate and disrupt our blood sugar levels and metabolism. The two tastes often become confused by our corrupted palate. We end up eating sugar and heavily-processed carbs that quickly break down into sugar to quench our thirst for natural, healthy fat.

Eat whatever looks shiny, bright and healthy: The brightest and shiniest food stuff now in the shops is likely to be man-made, genetically modified or artificially enhanced to fool us with its good looks. The instinct that used to guide us to the brightest, ripest fruit now drives us into the cereal aisles where the best packaging is to be found. This visual trickery is enhanced when companies spend thousands of pounds of research working out how to appeal to our subliminal instinctive urge to grab the thing that looks the most attractive.

Wake up when it's light and sleep when dark: The advent of artificial light entices us to stay awake late into the night allured by TV and the internet. Where once we slept long to survive the winter and short to feast on the bounty of summer, we now brazenly ignore the natural rhythm of the seasons to our detriment. Where we were once relaxed, rested and alert, many of us are now buzzing and 'wired' or dead on our feet.

Copy the posture and movement of these around us: Finally, our postures, once tall and proud, came from learning to squat, stand and move like our supreme athlete mothers and fathers – just how nature intended. Today, however, our naturally balanced bodies are contorted by modern furniture, sedentary living and the exaggerated swagger, stoop or gait of culturally prominent stereotypes promulgated by the mass media. Back pain and limited mobility are now typical among the young and old.

In short, our animal instincts simply won't work for us whilst we are blindly tempted, teased and ultimately betrayed by empty modern promises of physical and nutritional nourishment.

Compelling urges, that served us so well in antiquity, are now mistakenly doing us untold harm as we mistranslate them in a modern context. The pursuit of an easy life and the lures created by whole industries designed to tempt these basic human needs are compromising our looks, health and sometimes our sanity.

If you're not happy with your health, your body, your weight, your eating habits and your lack of exercise – IT'S NOT YOUR FAULT! Your instincts have been led astray. Like an unsuspecting fish hooked by a lure more appealing than its natural prey, we are all falling for the artificially attractive offerings served up not for our wellbeing, but for the wellbeing of profit-driven big business.

All those unhealthy habits you could not understand (and which have not been serving you well up until this point) have simply been the folly of your best intentioned instincts. However, once you know what's going on you can see these false idols for what they really are. You can draw a line in the sand and start again, aware of these hard-wired instincts and taking them into account to make better choices in future. Thus you can immunise yourself against the constant traps that the modern world lays out in wait for us.

Consciously and intelligently, you can develop the ability to let your instincts work for you and not against you. The healthier your body gets, the clearer the signal it gives your brain about what you really need right now. If you are getting injuries, ailments or sickness, that's your body telling you something. Ultimately, that's what the rest of this book is about: getting in touch with your real needs, your true instincts; the deeper, subtle shades of feeling that all too often get drowned out by the blare of commercial advertising, the artificiality of modern tastes, the desire for a quick food-fix, or the dream of a magic bullet.

Our unchangeable human instincts can be re-harnessed to new healthy habits, based on the ways of living for which we are evolutionarily best adapted.

> *If the* **TEN BASIC HUMAN INSTINCTS** *ring true for you, read on and find out how you can allow them to serve you and reach a level of fitness and health you never knew possible.*

Finally I'm going to introduce you to the three principles that make up the nuts and bolts of Instinctive Fitness ('IF' I'll sometimes call it for convenience). You'll learn more about each as we go on. Later in the book each aspect has a dedicated chapter.

1. **Natural Food**
2. **Natural Movement** *(including natural posture)*
3. **Natural Living**

IF says that if you can make improvements in any one of these areas you're on your way to a happier, healthier life. But if you can become proficient in, or even fully master, all of these areas, the results you'll experience will surpass your highest expectations.

When done the IF way, these elements come together with a potency that changes everything. It results in a wholly new life – one that works seamlessly, feels right and provides tangible benefits that reinforce the value of these new behaviours.

The upcoming chapters will deal with each of these factors in greater depth, but before we get to those I think I need to explain why there seems to be a need for a book to tell people what 'natural' means in these contexts.

You might think *anything* that human beings do is natural because we are inescapably part of nature - and you're right. *However*, while some actions, movements and foods are in line with the way that our bodies and minds evolved to work best, others most definitely are not. Our environment has changed so fast that we have not evolved fast enough to keep up (for reasons we'll look at later). The story of how we departed from this time-tested blueprint for the good life is fascinating, controversial and extraordinary – as the next few chapters will reveal.

Key Chapter points

- *Follow all the rules like I used to, and you probably still won't get the body you desire.*

- *Modern humans no longer live the lives that they evolved to lead. The instincts that we relied on for millennia are now devoid of the environment that made them useful.*

- *We don't need something 'new' to fight heart disease, obesity and diabetes; we can simply look back into our past and re-discover what made our ancient ancestors supremely fit, healthy and disease free!*

- *If you're not happy with your health, your body, your weight, your eating habits or your lack of exercise – it's not your fault! Your best instincts are being hijacked by insidious commercial forces and health and fitness propaganda.*

- *We can realign our Stone Age drives with the stimulation, challenges and nutrition that our bodies evolved to thrive on.*

- *We also need to immunise our minds from modern industries that contrive to ensnare us in the illusion of fulfilment.*

References:

1. Eaton SB, Konner M, Shostak M (1988) "Stone agers in the fast lane: chronic degenerative diseases in evolutionary perspective." American Journal of Medicine, 84:739-749.

"Medical anthropologists have found little cancer in their studies of technologically primitive people, and paleopathologists believe that the prevalence of malignancy was low in the past, even when differences in population age structure are taken into account" (Rowling, 1961; Hildes and Schaefer, 1984; Micozzi, 1991)

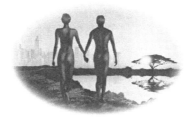

CHAPTER TWO

Truth, Falsehood and a 2.5 Million Year Experiment!

"A crank is a man with a new idea
- until it catches on"

Mark Twain

I wrote this book because I discovered that when you know the 10 human urges, a great physique and explosive energy are much simpler to achieve than we've been led to believe. For years we've been swallowing the pack of lies that fitness requires hardship, work and starvation. I can't think of any other area so important to all our lives, yet so swamped with preconceived and harmful notions – notions which actually jeopardise the dream of achieving real fitness, perfect health and a deep sense of wellbeing.

The sad fact is that although many people *are* initially prepared to pursue their personal fitness goals against their innate nature, they simply don't have the time or the will to question whether what they are being told is correct – or whether these opinions dressed up as fact might actually be doing them more harm than good.

Knowing the 10 human urges makes life simpler

On the following page are seven of the commonest fallacies that wreck our chances of success right from the outset, and damage our instinct for what is good for us.

The Seven Fallacies of Modern Fitness

- *There are no good results without serious EFFORT: There's no gain without pain.*

- *Exercise can't be enjoyable for itself - overcoming pain and discomfort is part of the process.*

- *Exercise should leave you pretty tired because it has to be stressful for the body to adapt and improve.*

- *Exercise (jogging, swimming, gym, etc) is a great way to keep your weight down.*

- *You need to diet for weight loss – eating less and avoiding fat is the best way.*

- *You need to accept that you're going to start going downhill from your 20s onwards. Old age and immobility creeps up on us from early in our lives and we just have to accept it.*

- *Some illnesses just HAPPEN. All you can do is eat sensibly ('a balanced diet'), do some moderately intense exercise 3 or 4 times a week, and hope for the best.*

As you read on, it's going to become steadily clearer why all of these pillars of Conventional Wisdom are utter hogwash, are damaging you, harming society and are doing the health and wealth of this country and others a serious disservice.

My aim over the coming pages is to convince you that the accepted science peddled by successive governments and the established media as a whole has been fundamentally flawed for years. When just the facts are placed under the microscope without the background of damaging pre-conceived opinion, they *demand* we rethink the way we look at ourselves, the way we treat our bodies and the way we look at fitness and health as a whole. Ultimately, who you listen to and the path you choose to take is going to impact both your own life and the lives of any future generations for which you have responsibility.

Introducing... an alternative 'truth'

For years now we have been led to believe by the media that we are all in need of a product, a service or endless advice on how to get ourselves into tip top form. We have stopped thinking about and, most importantly, 'feeling' what our bodies need to be fit and healthy. On top of this never-ending barrage of information on the best way to eat, drink and exercise, there is a continual stream of invasive advertising pouring into our consciousness that all contains a sub text: you need to buy or do something to be healthy and happy.

Instinctive Fitness encourages you to stop listening to what you are told and to start listening to what your body tells you and let your instincts lead the way.

IF's Five Truths of Modern Living

1. *This background noise of modern living means that nearly all of us have* **lost the instinct for what's best for us.** *We have overcomplicated a subject (Health and Fitness) that should be so simple that we do the right things* **instinctively.** *All we need to do to regain proper health and fitness is to listen closely to these instincts and align ourselves with their original intention. We don't need to burrow further into text books and magazines for answers, or indeed to surround ourselves with fancy gyms or experts.*

2. *Exercise should be a de-stressing experience, not traumatic or involving much psychological effort. If you are stressing about exercise: "Am I doing in right, am I doing enough" or if you're simply not enjoying it – you <u>are</u> doing something wrong.*

3. *Health and body composition are easily fixed when we start eating good food. Eating the right food starts with buying the right food; and buying the right food means ignoring the 'bait foods' put out to tempt us.*

4. *Physical weakness and frailty comes about largely through our own neglect and misuse of the bodies we have been given. The 'use it or lose it' principle applies to at least 85% of our lost physical capacity in old age, with only the remaining 15% actually attributable to the time we have spent alive. Much pain and discomfort simply arises through doing things our bodies shouldn't be doing. If we stop doing these things, the pain (which was trying to tell us something) melts away.*

5. *Our genetic programming dictates that we can and should be active, vibrant and well right up to the last days of our long, long lives. A slow, drawn-out decline is, on the most part, not inevitable.*

How can I claim these things?

Of course any claim should be backed up with sound scientific evidence, and the good news is that we already *have* the clear indisputable results in form an on-going experiment that has been running for the last 2.5 million years – in fact the total amount of time that hominids have walked the earth. *(I've also included more references to scientific papers that I think you will get through... but let me know if you run out!)*

It's now vital that we look at the results of the world's longest running, most comprehensively researched, undisputable experiment ever undertaken; an experiment that cannot be credibly ridiculed or challenged by any so called 'expert' – because *this* experiment has been carried out by an authority higher than any modern institution: nature itself.

The 2.5 Million Year Experiment and Our Supreme Ancestors

What I was stunned to find out in researching my personal transformation is that our ancient 'hunter-gatherer' ancestors were not in any way lacking in health, but were in fact exceptionally strong, fit people who, assuming they successfully avoided accidents, infections and predators, lived long active lives. I discovered a wealth of solid **scientific evidence**[1] that proved not only this, but also that they suffered from almost <u>none</u> of the modern diseases (the so-called 'diseases of civilisation') with which modern society currently wrestles.

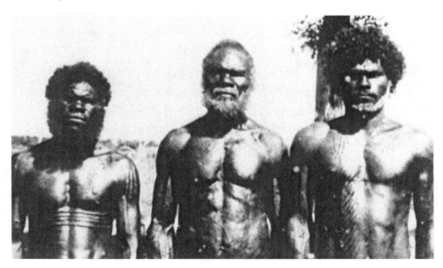

For 99% of the time this experiment has been running, humans lived nomadic lives, roaming the plains and forests, surviving on what they could hunt and forage. Contrary to the common misconception that early man lived a 'nasty, brutish and short' life (as Thomas Hobbes famously wrote); archaeological bone records demonstrate quite the opposite. Indeed, anthropologists who study the human form are united in their view that 'primitive humans' (i.e. most humans that have ever lived) were in fact strong, lean, agile and healthy creatures who often enjoyed lives as long as those we do today.[2]

Although hunter-gatherers' *average* life expectancy was quite low in comparison to ours, this was caused mainly by a high percentage dying in childbirth, and of accidents and infection – all of which seriously skew the statistics. Those that did survive these hazards frequently lived into their 70s. In other words, they had life spans that were comparable with our own. And this was, of course, in the days before the NHS offered free medical care to extend people's lives well past the point that nature would otherwise let them perish.

As these early people didn't have the benefit of drugs, medical treatment or social services to sustain life, we can safely assume that they would have been reasonably active and healthy right up until their final days. In fact, *only* if they were active and healthy would they have stood a chance of surviving in the continuously mobile nature of the nomadic lifestyle.

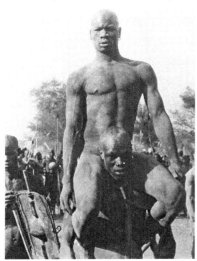
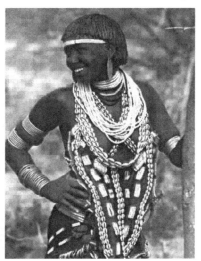

The rot sets in

However, 10,000 years ago, when the obvious allure of **agriculture** took over as a way of life – just a few minutes ago in evolutionary terms – records clearly show that humans quickly became shorter, weaker and frailer; started suffering from a whole host of never before seen diseases; and started living much shorter lives.

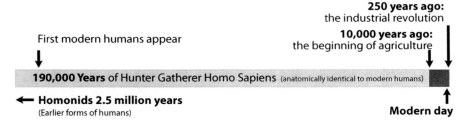

This new, modern farmer typically died in their thirties – even the Egyptian Pharaohs (who didn't personally do much farming but who lived off its bounty) fared no better, and they lacked for nothing! The evidence shows very clearly that the decision to remain in one place and farm the land had, for reasons we will cover later, a seriously detrimental effect on the health of our species.[3]

> *As far-out as this may sound, it's really not the product of fanciful thinking. Please check out the references throughout the book which link to the scientific papers that bear these facts out. See especially: "Longevity among Hunter-Gatherers: A cross cultural examination," by Guven M, and Kaplan H (2007)*

These new agriculturally-dependent humans suddenly became prone to a rash of new diseases, the like of which still plague us today despite the advances of modern science. Of course farmers, which most humans essentially were at this time, still led pretty active lifestyles, but their life spans were already seriously compromised by the introduction of new food types, such as previously indigestible grains like wheat, maize and corn that were made edible through the invention of new processing methods.

Because it was far easier to produce rather than gather, food supply became more plentiful. With more dependable quantities, the use of agriculture to sustain us expanded to a massive scale. Since it was now possible to feed people in numbers previously unthinkable, populations began to grow – fast. The food stuffs the new grains replaced, of course, were meat and vegetables, which could no longer be sourced in the local area in enough quantity to provide for these fast growing numbers; so, as a species we became increasingly more dependent on the crops cultivated around us.

Modern consequences

Today, thousands of years later, following an industrial *and* a technological revolution, we are chained more than ever to eating these essentially inedible foods in ever greater quantities – and so are suffering ever more from the fact that these foods are intrinsically indigestible to humans (as is born out with the growing phenomena of so called 'intolerances'). Moreover, not only is our food processed on an industrial scale, but we no longer even have to keep our bodies active – to a great extent compounding the original nutritional shortfall!

So here we are today, with an abundance of readily available, cheap and usually sugar-filled food *and* redundant from physical activity: we can sit in office chairs or cars for much of the day, free from the need for any type of physical labour. Therefore, in addition to these harmful new foods we shovel into our mouths, we've now added an equally harmful sedentary pattern of living, and pay the 'double whammy' price for this 'easy existence' every day.

The price we are all paying for agriculture on a massive industrial scale and easy-to-come-by food means that the growing number of us occupying the modern world you and I know so well are now paying the biggest price – being the flabbiest, slowest, least healthy humans ever to have walked the earth!

10,000 years on, we humans have still barely started to evolve to deal with these comparatively new practices of eating and living: we make our livelihoods solely with our brains (rather than our bodies) and essentially consume naturally innutritious foods made tolerably consumable in factories. You see, when human evolution is viewed in its proper context, we are effectively still Stone Age humans, composed of Stone Age genes demanding Stone Age conditions. These genes *expect* to engage with the pressures and resources of a Stone Age environment. In many areas where we have departed from this ideal genetic blueprint, the gap between our actual lives and the life our genes evolved to deal with is filled with disease, pain, immobility and unhappiness.

It's a Caveman's life

In contrast to today's lifestyle, our pre-agricultural ancestors enjoyed a high level of fitness and health throughout their lives, achieved through eating the foods nature provided for them and performing the daily tasks needed for survival. However, this was far from a full-time job, leaving plenty of time for relaxation, play and time with their family and tribe.

So although they did have to cope with the fact that they could never take their next meal or day-to-day survival for granted, they did get to lead vibrant, energetic and healthy lives, filled with plenty of time for fun, games, celebrations, storytelling and laughter. In fact they enjoyed lives that an increasing number of members of this modern 'stressed out' society would be truly envious of today, even if they never had the modern technology and all the apparent advantages it brings us.

More and more of this mounting evidence tells the story, not of a poor hard-done-by creature, struggling to scratch out a wretched existence, but of a healthy, intelligent and resourceful creature, living what many in this stressful modern world would consider closer to an idyllic lifestyle.

'Noble Savage' or Captain Caveman?

Why is it that we blindly accept the stereotypical image of a brutish, stupid caveman with his club, hunched stance and grunted speech, dragging his woman back to the cave by the hair?

When primitive humans first became widely known about from 18th Century fossil discoveries they were initially revered for their purity of purpose and spirit. They were seen as 'noble savages' by pioneering philosophers such as Jean-Jacques Rousseau. However, once Darwin's Theory of Evolution became more accepted in late 19th century, the prudish Victorians simply couldn't accept that they could be related to such an unwashed primitive creature.

So in their wisdom, they decided instead to do what only a proper upstanding Englishman *could* do: deny the truth and rebrand the caveman as an utter philistine who could never be any relation to a gentleman – let alone their dainty but up-tight, corset wearing queen.

Even today this thuggish stereotype perpetuates, and even your author has to resist the well-conditioned temptation to conjure up images of a stooped, grunting, bearskin-wearing oaf when the word 'caveman' is uttered.

This is just the same sort of 'rebranding' that happened to Father Christmas.

Picture Father Christmas in your head, right now. If you have in your mind's eye a tubby chap with a red suit on, with a white beard and great big sack of parcels, you're not picturing some legend handed down over centuries from generation to generation – but actually an image popularised by a culturally pervasive 1930s ad campaign by Coca Cola.

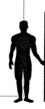

So as I have asked before in this book, and I'll surely ask again: please put your clichéd, long-held conceptions of what cavemen were like to one side for the next few minutes while I re-acquaint you with our fit, agile, healthy, magnificent ancient relatives.

A day in a nomadic life

Numerous studies suggest that on average our hunter-gatherer ancestors would spend between 2-4 hours a day foraging or hunting for food. This would involve plenty of walking, some intermittent light jogging, jumping, bending, climbing, squatting, cutting, throwing, lifting, carrying and other basic human movements.

Inevitably, on occasion, they would have put in very short bursts of effort to sprint after their prey or to avoid becoming prey themselves. However, it was vital for their survival that they were able to recover from these efforts almost instantly to ensure they were not in a weakened state to meet a passing sabre toothed tiger or giant bear.

This meant that, except in occasional dire circumstance,
our ancestors would never have chosen to push themselves
through the pain barrier unless they had no option.

Although they knew all too well how to manage their bodies and their energy expenditure, they certainly wouldn't have consciously analysed or endlessly stressed over the best way to keep in shape. They would have achieved their supreme fitness *easily* and without any special method or consideration. It simply flowed out of their lifestyle; essentially a birthright, not something they needed to strive for.

Dietary choices were in fact simple. When they caught or found any edible food they ate it immediately, or carried it back to the camp to feed their tribe. They ate whatever was available in the season and (unless it can be proven otherwise) no antelope ever came with a label showing the amount of sugar, carbohydrate or saturated fat it contained. However, far from spurning the fatty cuts for the leaner meat, they would surely have prized and probably squabbled over animal fat when they had the opportunity – as a prime source of fuel it would have been one of the most prized parts of the animal.

In a world without sugar, processed carbohydrates and seductive packaging, they certainly never felt the need to count calories or worry about making good dietary choices. In other words, they did the things that came *naturally* to them and that they needed to do to survive.

If they gave their body composition any special thought at all, their instinct would have been to try to *put on weight* to guard against the possibility of any future famines. The foods they ate and their active lives meant that, although they were often able to eat until they were full, putting on additional body fat was easier said than done.

Finally – and this might come as a shock to you – at a time where there was no health advice, no blood tests and certainly no fish oil capsules or beta-blockers...

> *...our ancient ancestors hardly suffered from any obesity, diabetes, high cholesterol, stress, high blood pressure, heart-disease or any forms of cancer at all!* [4]

The evidence from modern 'ancient' tribes

Anthropologists are continually updating us with fresh evidence from bones and a variety of other archaeological evidence on our ancient hunter-gatherer forefathers, but this is far from the only source of information that attests to how they lived their very different lives. Today there are many contemporary tribes still living on the fringes of our modern world, and although compressed into smaller and smaller spaces and continually challenged by interference from the outside world, many still live a healthy and happy existence – while all around them our so-called 'civilised world' increasingly struggles with its own, home-grown health epidemic.

Present-day hunter-gatherers like the Hiwi, Hadza, Ache and !Kung groups, with no access to modern medical care whatsoever, have plenty of members who make it well into their 80s – a feat that the UK was only able to boast long after the creation of the National Health Service.

For these tribal members, however, this is nothing special – nor has it ever been. Despite a lifelong struggle for food, shelter and clothing, many of these so-called primitive tribes enjoy great health to a ripe old age.

So would it not be safe to use these people as our guide to better health? What kind of lives could we lead if we followed their lead and merely *bolstered* our health with modern health care? Is it not safe to assume that our ancient ancestors enjoyed similar good health to these modern tribes? After all, they knew an unmolested, bountiful prehistoric world rich in flora and fauna. Is it not arrogant and misguided to presume that our forbearers who enjoyed a world free from pollution were either physically or mentally inferior to us? Roaming in what we today would consider unimaginable space, how daft would we look to them; all sickly, weak and cooped up in our polluted, carved up, fenced in modern environment?

It is my hope that you will choose to exchange an array of outworn ideas that have been holding us back for centuries with a new instinct for living that expresses the maximum potential inherent in being a human animal.

Why is Instinctive Fitness different?

For the past 50 years, while the western world's health has rapidly declined, we have been continuously bombarded with theories and opinions about what makes us fit and healthy – but what most people don't realise (even though it's clear that we *are* getting steadily less healthy) is that the vast majority of the information we are given as fact is absolute bunk: useless or worse than useless.

The Instinctive Fitness system offers something genuinely new – not just a few exercises to be repeated until bored or a restrictive Spartan diet to be followed to the letter.

You really <u>can</u> totally transform your body without extended efforts, low-calorie dieting, endless repetitions, boring cardio or wasted time at the gym.

What we've developed is a whole lifestyle programme which, although less strict and regimented than any fad diet you may have tried, does follow a few radical, but life-changing rules. It involves changing the way you think about key aspects of your life as a whole, and openly questions much of the perceived wisdom of our age. If you don't think you're open-minded enough to swim against this unrelenting tide of opinion, please return this book to the shelf right now to remain as firmly closed as your mind.

Still here? Great! The Instinctive Fitness approach tends to take over people's thinking until they have their lives and their bodies just the way they want them. One of my clients called it a 'benign cult' the other day, which made me laugh. I think he was getting at the way that, if you let it, the programme alters the way you see health and fitness forever. It's true though: this isn't just about training people, it's about putting them back in touch with their true physical nature.

Instinctive Fitness isn't about placing even more burdens onto an already stressful existence. It's about letting fitness develop and grow naturally and organically. It's about stress free *play* and eating the best gourmet food – not enduring calorie counted deprivation.

The Key Points of Instinctive Fitness

- *Superior health, not just superior fitness. Lots of programmes actually sacrifice health in a misinformed attempt to maximise short-term fitness gains.*

- *You'll eat in a totally different way to the usual faddy, restrictive plans that you've come across before. We won't even ask you to try to eat less. You'll eat like a gourmet, not a mouse.*

- *You won't need to push yourself hard to get fit. You won't be pushing any pain barriers or training like you're going for SAS selection. Boot camp is out! So are hours on a stationary bike. It won't take up hour after hour of your time every week.*

- *Learning the principles of 'Instinctive Fitness' is fascinating in itself, as I hope you'll agree as you read the rest of the book. For everything I recommend, I explain the reason for it based on research and logic, not personal opinion or whimsy.*

- *It's a programme that anyone can do, regardless of age, gender or how fit or unfit they are.*

- *It's a programme about maximising pleasure in your life, not pain. You shouldn't need the discipline of a Benedictine monk to stick with this. That's why it can, and should, be a* **programme for life** *– not a ridiculously dishonest '3-weeks-to-a-six-pack' approach.*

Lee

Lee, 40, was my very first personal training client to try out my 30-day programme. When we first met he told me that he couldn't understand why he wasn't feeling as great as he should; after all, he worked outdoors all day long as a landscape gardener. I pointed out that although he worked hard and burnt a lot of calories, he was still getting out of breath quite quickly with only minor exertion and that he shouldn't be totally exhausted at the end of the day.

It was sad to hear him tell me how this late afternoon energy flag left him with little interest in pursuing an active life outside his work on week days, and avoiding anything too strenuous at the weekend in case he ran out of puff doing the day job the next week. This left Lee feeling rather trapped in a lifestyle – existing to work rather than working to enjoy life.

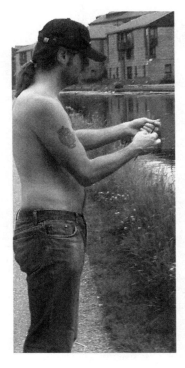

But the final straw came as he got increasingly embarrassed about the paunch around his midriff - to the point he no longer wanted to take his top off in the summer!

I ran him through the regime I'd been following to see what he thought, and suggested that, even though he was active in his day job, plodding away for hours in his garden work might be the cause of some of his problem. He was suffering from low energy *because* of this continual slow pace, and what he needed was a mixture of short, sharp, high-intensity movement thrown into the mix to bring some back some of his old zap. I put together an exercise programme that complimented Lee's normal lifestyle and daily routine and helped him to stick to it for just 30 days.

Lee was also eating what conventional wisdom would tell you is a reasonable diet: not too much red meat and plenty of high energy foods, such as bread, pasta, potatoes and rice. He had been led to believe that eating lots of what are commonly accepted as 'good' carbs was the key to having bags of energy, so he ate more, not understanding why they were failing to provide him with the energy he needed.

It took a little while for Lee to adapt to the new style of mixed intensity exercise that I was guiding him through, but, although initially sceptical, he went with it. He was also fascinated by the new way of eating I had proposed. Always strong in character, he committed to the eating plan right away and followed it pretty much to the letter from day one.

About 2 weeks into our 30-day pro-gramme, after only 4 exercise sessions, I remember him ringing me in total amazement, flabbergasted by what was happening to his body:

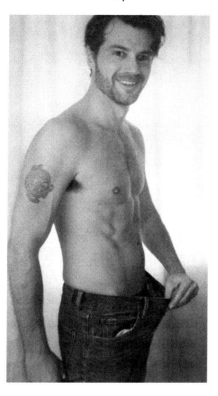

"Olly, I've not lost much weight yet but – you're not going to believe this – I've had to tighten my belt by three notches!"

Actually, it was easy for *me* to believe. Lee's stomach had become swollen with the consumption of the wrong kinds of food, but when he had a break from them, the gaseous bloating started to subside immediately, leaving him three inches slimmer around the waist.

Lee saw such fantastic results during my 30 day trial he stuck with me and just four months later he had lost over 10kg, could see each abdominal muscle and possessed a powerful physique that most men would kill for. But he didn't do this with masses of self-discipline and abstinence - in fact he ate like a king and he always looked forward to our workouts!

Every day he rewarded himself for his long days gardening with beautifully-cooked roasts accompanied by lashings of vegetables. He always ate until 'full' (or sometimes 'stuffed'), and never deprived himself of calories, and the best bit is all his meal choices contained ingredients worthy of the very best Michelin-starred restaurants.

He says he now knows how to lose weight 'on demand' and on the odd occasion he's been lured back to the dark side on high days and holidays with family or friends, it just made him feel dreadful. In Lee's own words:

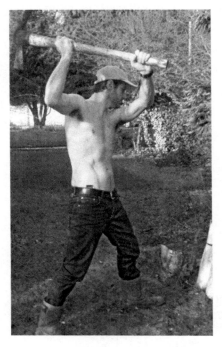

"I still find it hard to believe a diet so widely accepted as the optimal could make me feel so bad!"

He now gets home in the evening to eat a deliciously satisfying, sizeable meal and then decides where to unleash the bountiful energy he still has at his disposal.

It might sound too good to be true, but Lee and many others are happy to contradict anyone who says fitness can't happen this way. To hear Lee talk more about his transformation, visit **www.instinctive-fitness.com/ testimonials**. He'll tell you how he's stuck with this way of eating, moving and living – and how he can't ever see this changing. (Most 'dieters', by contrast, are back to their old weight and old habits in a matter of months!)

I don't think you need to read too far between the lines to understand the life-changing impact the Instinctive Fitness programme has had on Lee; and, happily, he's not an exception to the rule. From experience, I can confidently predict that simply by sticking to the Instinctive Fitness programme for just 30 days, you too can start to achieve these same sorts of results; no matter what your current starting point, age or gender.

These methods work just as well for women, if not better. The following 'before and after' photo of Leigh, a student at Edinburgh University, shows why women needn't worry that they will put on muscle through the brief, occasional amount of strength work that the programme includes. (No, I don't only train people called Lee/Leigh!)

I think you'll agree Leigh's transformation is stunning, but it's also informative. She didn't include much more exercise than daily walks to aid her transformation. I advise more exercise than this (for total, all-round fitness) but it shows how getting your diet right is the foundation of all future success.

Spreading the word

Working with individuals was great, and the personal rewards were fantastic – getting paid to keep fit myself while watching my clients transform in front of my very eyes was a buzz, but I soon realised that I was only going to have an impact on a very few people, and something more ambitious was needed if I was to spread the word wider. A new approach was required if I was to pass this precious hidden knowledge on to *all* the people in the world who, like me, desperately needed it.

Nowadays, through my *Instinctive Fitness Programme* I have the privilege to have a radical impact on people's lives, transforming their physiques, health, wellbeing, and athletic potential. I raise awareness of the truth behind the lies we've been sold through interviews, articles and the internet. I now help people from all over to start tapping into the power of our lost ancestry with my popular free **30-day transformation package** that can be found at **www.instinctive-fitness.com.**

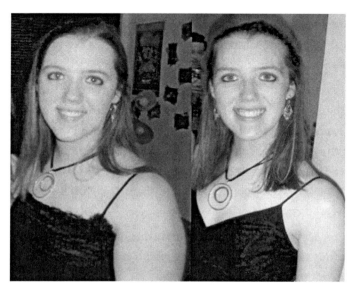

At IF we gather the combined wisdom from many expert sources to provide a one-stop resource to start living a life that honours the instincts and inheritance of the natural health we all already possess. It provides not just advice and ideas to help people to re-discover their entitlement to be fit and healthy but, most importantly, offers a completely new mental approach to health and fitness. We remove the burden of forced exercise and restricted diets, and go back to using our bodies as they were intended: eating, sleeping and playing without target weights or performance goals, and certainly without added pressure or guilt.

All things considered...

I believe the shameful way that we've been led to believe our physical prowess is beyond our control in the media, through TV, and via 'big business' advertising which implies we are in some way 'broken', has left us feeling confused, paranoid and desperate for new answers. Naively, we listen to anyone who shouts loudly enough offering us the latest new wonder product/diet or super food.

As a society, we have been conditioned to consider ourselves weak, flawed and in need of some kind of outside assistance, but we're not and we don't, and I aim to prove to you that every one of us has far more potential than we may ever dare dream. I promise to reintroduce you to the real truth that stands before you if you can suspend your current beliefs and look once again at your body through the indisputably wise eyes of your ancestors.

But don't accept the ideas I offer blindly; please question them, think about them – but ultimately allow your *instinct* to tell you whether your ancestors were right all along. These ideas and concepts may inspire you or they may invoke a hostile reaction - but ultimately the choice of whether you choose to give them a try is yours – if you don't, it really doesn't matter what you think of the theory, as you'll never know if it would work for you.

Are you ready to hear an alternative truth: an ancient truth which tells us fitness does come naturally? A truth which enables health and wellness to blossom without effort or stress?

Instinctive Fitness means you no longer need listen to all those experts who'd have you believe you're not in control of your body; you no longer need to heed the wisdom that convinces you that you're powerless. This is an opportunity for you to retake command and mastership of your body *and* mind to unleash your magnificent 'caveperson' within!

Key Chapter Points:

This chapter has made the case that we should realign ourselves with these powerful instincts nature provided for us with a new vision, logical thinking, and some new habits. We can get back on our evolutionary path, the true road to becoming our best possible selves.

- *Don't believe something just because it's commonly accepted. The health and fitness industry is founded on 7 wasteful, sometimes damaging, fallacies.*

- *Our knowledge of human evolution is the perfect guide to staying fit and well, as this experiment has been running for 2.5 million years.*

- *After 10,000 years, humans have still not evolved to new practices such as making a living solely with our brains and eating heavily-processed foods.*

- *If we learn to appreciate the bare facts of our evolutionary past and the reason for our evolutionary drives, we can restore an instinct for optimum performance and healthful living that has been lost through insidiously harmful modern trends.*

References:

1. Dunn FL (1968) "Epidemiological factors: health and disease in hunter-gatherers." In: Man the Hunter, eds. Lee RB, DeVore I; Aldine Publishing, Chicago, pp. 221-228.

2. Guven M, Kaplan H (2007) "Longevity among Hunter-Gatherers: A cross cultural examination." [Online] Available at: http://www.anth.ucsb.edu/faculty/gurven/papers/pdrdraft04182006.pdf

3. Ho K-J, et al. (1971) "Studies on the Masai." Archeological Pathology, 91:387; Mann GV, et al. (1972) "Atherosclerosis in the Maasai." American Journal of Epidemiology, 95:26-37

4. Dr. Richard G. Cutler, molecular gerontologist and longevity expert from the US National Institute for Ageing, estimates that, based on laboratory analysis of skeletal remains, the "maximum lifespan potential" of Homo Sapiens of 15,000 years ago was 91 years of age.

Carerra-Bastos P, Fontes-Villalba M, O'Keefe JH et al. (2011) "The western diet and lifestyle and diseases of civilization." [Online] Available at: http://dx.doi.org/10.2147/RRCC.S16919, 15-35

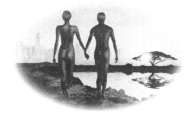

CHAPTER THREE

From Bad to Worse

"It isn't that they can't see the solution.

It is that they can't even see the problem"

G.K. Chesterton

In this short chapter I'm going to briefly sum up the current situation with regard to the UK's health. If you're anywhere else in the western world reading this, the story is pretty much the same and just as painful to read.

> If you're ready to give the Instinctive Fitness approach a try and to get straight to the nitty-gritty, you could skip to Chapter Six where I explain the IF approach to eating and diet. However, if you want the full picture and the full motivation to push through with the master plan, I recommend reading the book straight through, so you see how the whole jigsaw fits together.

Is the NHS getting it wrong?

Medical care has continued to improve in all kinds of ways over recent decades and many diseases that might have killed us thirty years ago can now be easily cured with new treatments. This can only be good, but it does reflect a continued bias of the medical community towards *treating* diseases rather than *preventing* them in the first place.

Only with an emphasis on long-term, on-going measures to prevent physical decline, promote health and stave off disease – rather than just *problem fixing* – will we be able to prevent expensive future medical intervention being required so frequently and increase the quality of life for a whole nation.

The medical establishment has, in my opinion, been too focused from day one on treating symptoms rather than looking for and heading off the underlying causes of poor health.

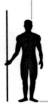

Thomas Edison (1847 – 1931, who held the patent for the first incandescent light) has not yet been proved right when he said: "The doctor of the future will give no medicine, but will interest her or his patients in the care of the human frame, in a proper diet, and in the cause and prevention of disease".

Although we are becoming ever better at patching people up once they have a health problem, it has to be acknowledged that modern disease continues to run rampant. Here are a few bald statistics:[1]

- *1 in 2 men will be diagnosed with cancer at some point in their lives (with the figure for women not much better).*

- *As many as 1 in 3 deaths this year will be from heart disease.*

- *7 out of 10 adults have high blood pressure. Even half of under 35s have an unhealthy level, (according to a report by Lloyd's Pharmacy in Feb 2012)*

- *Obesity, which is the 5th leading risk factor for global deaths, is a growing problem (no pun intended) and has doubled across the world since 1980. Almost one in four adults in England was classified as obese in 2009. 44% of men and 33% of women were classified as overweight in the same year.*

- *The obesity situation for children is even more worrying. Despite their youth, 3 in 10 children under 15 were also classified as overweight or obese in 2009. In the same year, only 1 in 5 children were found to be eating 5 portions of vegetables a day.*

For adults and children an increased BMI (Body Mass Index) is a major risk factor for:

- *cardiovascular diseases (mainly heart disease and stroke, the leading cause of death in 2009)*
- *diabetes;*
- *musculoskeletal disorders (especially osteoarthritis - a highly disabling degenerative disease of the joints);*
- *some cancers (especially endometrial, breast, and colon).*

In short: if you are carrying too much body fat, take your head out of the sand and act now!

It's not about avoiding saturated fat!

Almost everybody thinks fat makes you fat. This simple misunderstanding results in a population struggling and failing to lose weight.

The figures bear this out. During 2008/09, **people in the UK were eating less saturated fat than at any point in the past.** In fact we've generally been studiously doing exactly what we've been told to for decades. We were told that we were fat because we ate too much fat (admittedly, there's a misleading sense of intuitive logic there), and the British public has vilified this natural food source for the last half century.

However, the point that can't be avoided any longer is that, despite our general compliance with the government's health advice, obesity shows no signs of doing anything other than becoming *more* common.

We have to accept it: **we have been given the wrong advice**. The prescription we have been given is wrong. It's been tried, tested and found wanting.

It's simply *not* an excess of fat making us, as a nation, horribly overweight. As much as it's healthy to avoid some particular types of dangerous fat, **it is in fact, the consumption of processed, energy-dense, nutrient-light *carbohydrate* that is driving the obesity epidemic.**

"Preposterous" I hear you cry, *"how can you condone the consumption of saturated fat and warn of the dangers of our beloved whole grains"?*

I beg you to suspend everything you've been told up to now, and look at the evidence...

The Inuits

For thousands of years the native population of what is now called Alaska lived on a diet consisting almost entirely of animal fat. For generations they consumed the fat of seals and walruses with no heart disease, no diabetes and no obesity! In the latter part of the last century with new communication channels and trade coming into their remote homeland, western ideology and products started being adopted into their lifestyles.

Over this period a new generation has grown up ever more reliant on carbohydrate-rich foods containing wheat and sugar, and the Inuit now find themselves joining in the sad decline that the UK and much of the rest of the western world has experienced.

Even though the UK's total calorific intake has fallen since 2006, its consumption of complex carbohydrates and its waistlines have grown hand in hand. Our increasing dependence on bread, potatoes and pasta to feed our fast food lifestyles in preference to healthy meats and vegetables is strong evidence for the fact that focussing all our attention on lowering the consumption of fat and eating fewer calories does not lead to *sustained* body fat loss.

Perversely our modern thinking on food has created another side to the obesity coin. Anorexia and bulimia are two serious conditions of malnutrition brought about by a low-calorie intake. Our obsession with diet, exercise and body shape is breeding an unhealthy attitude to eating and a misjudged emphasis on thinness over health. Those touting the blinkered low fat/low-calorie message have to look at the evidence before their eyes and take responsibility for its dangerous extremes.

Get up and move!

Another issue is that of immobility. With an ageing population, the number of people who lose their mobility only continues to grow. Lack of mobility is not only a massive problem for those who suffer from not being able to get about – doing chores, the shopping, socialising and generally having a good time – but it also massively increases the risk of almost every other disease we have already mentioned.

But don't be fooled, it's not just the old that are suffering. It's estimated that 4 out of 5 people in the UK will experience crippling back pain at some stage in their lives. (In parts of the less developed world this figure is more like 4 in 100!)

As a personal trainer, this sort of dysfunction comes as no surprise to me. I watch the way that people walk and move around on the streets of the UK and I note just how far they are from the natural posture that humans should display. Even when I see children walking to school, I see from their slouched postures that their athleticism will be severely compromised and that they are setting themselves up to become the hunched office workers of the future.

I see the results of people who spend all day sitting badly in chairs, gradually increasing the effect of gravity on their spine until they no longer have even one joint that has a proper range of movement. The chair-bound individual is then well on the path towards an old age in which he or she is bent over so far forwards that only pulling their head well back allows them to look straight ahead. Not a good look!

So what are we doing about this?

The NHS has developed treatments for dealing with some of these ailments and diseases as and when they present themselves. Doctors are given targets to meet, so they generally treat problems with drugs or surgery which usually alleviate the *symptoms,* but they aren't encouraged to spend any time thinking about preventative medicine or to take much time to consider the cause of the disease. Their training, while broad-ranging and diverse, includes barely a side-long glance at dietary factors, exercise and preventative medicine.

What we don't have is any sort of comprehensive system for ensuring that these problems never happen in the first place. Surely, as the saying goes, an ounce of prevention is worth a pound of cure?

At the risk of sounding too cynical, it has to be pointed out there is much more money to be made in treating diseases with fancy, expensive drugs than there is in establishing practices which keep disease (and dis-ease) at bay. There is no doubt that a preventative approach would save taxpayers' money in the long-run; however, fat-cat pharmaceutical companies would not find this development to be a profitable one."

One prong in any well organised programme – personal or national – is getting people moving again. This just isn't happening at the moment for adults or for children. Provision for school sport in the UK is weak because our political masters, in their wisdom, have sold off our playing fields and haven't left enough time for sports or play in an ever more crowded, target-driven curriculum.

National 'couch syndrome'

We have truly become a sedentary nation. In 2008, only 39% of men and 29% of women met the government's recommendation of 2 ½ hours of exercise a week. Less than a quarter of adults now play regular sport ('regular' defined as more than 11 occasions per month). Over 44% of men are sedentary for more than 6 hours a day at weekends. (The figures for women are little better.)

"If it weren't for the fact that the TV set and the refrigerator are so far apart, some of us wouldn't get any exercise at all."

Joey Adam (US comedian 1911-1999)

Even for those who do exercise during the week, the benefits they gain are often undermined by poor exercise selection. Most who choose a sport to keep fit fail to recognise the one-sided nature of their chosen activity and the inherent disadvantages it poses. Two examples of this are cycling and walking.

Cycling is often touted as great all-round exercise – but it's simply not. Cycling is great for the heart, lungs and leg muscles but is next to useless for improving posture, flexibility, agility, balance or upper body strength. Many cyclists have serious mobility issues that end up with a physio referral.

Even the benefits it does offer are quickly lost if the individual over-trains by pursuing the activity in the form of **heavy cardio**. A long, leisurely Sunday bike ride is great. Some quick hill sprints once or twice a week – even better. But logging hundreds of miles a week in a competitive frenzy where the intensity means you can no longer chat to your riding partner easily is a recipe for overtraining, exhaustion and compromised health. Pushed too hard, your body will react against all your efforts and intentions.

Another example: **walking** is fantastic exercise, working the body through chains of natural movement that have developed over millions of years. It's great basic aerobic exercise, inherently relaxing and it's easy on the joints. I'm going to say more about how fantastic it is later in the book. On its own though, it's only half a programme at best. To this will need to be added a number of different components, especially an element that involves working the body closer to its capacity for short periods of time.

Lift some weight

It is also essential that the body be challenged to lift heavier things every week (body-weight exercises can be sufficient) to ensure that strength continues to develop through your 30s, 40s and maybe even in your 50s. Thereafter, in later years, the aim is simply to hang onto as much strength and muscle mass as you can. Lean muscle mass has been shown to be an excellent indicator of future health and also reduces the risk of osteoporosis (the reduced bone density that often leads to fractures and brittle bones in old age).

The take home points of this section are that exercise needs to be a rounded affair with elements chosen judiciously to balance each other. Yes, it's important to do things you like and will stick with, but too many people have little understanding of the effect that their chosen sports or exercise has on their body – especially when taken to extremes or practised, like most of us, with a badly compressed spine.

As depressing as it sounds, my overall analysis of the situation is that most of us aren't doing enough and, of those of us who are, most do not have a balanced programme that promotes long-term development, injury avoidance and overall health.

The glum statistics we started the chapter with are caused by, in my opinion, a number of key factors:

- *Successive governments' well-meaning attempts to control our macronutrient balance (our dietary balance of calories from fat, carbs or protein) under pressure from lobby groups and industry.*

- *A food industry quick to capitalise on producing foods we crave – but which are often doing us untold harm.*

- *A medical industry more interested in dispensing drugs, under the guidance (and financial support) of the pharmaceutical industry than actually finding the underlying causes.*

- *A pharmaceutical industry focused on the profit from selling drugs to the medical industry.*

- *A general lifestyle that is almost devoid of the sort of movement we need to remain properly functioning human beings.*

So as you can see, there is no other person or organisation of influence that you can trust to have your best interests as their number one consideration. The fact is, the only person with responsibility over your overall health and wellbeing is YOU.

Key Chapter Points:

- *Modern diseases are becoming more common, despite medical advances in other areas.*

- *Heart disease, obesity, diabetes, cancer, stress and depression are rampant, although these diseases were totally unknown to our ancient predecessors.*

- *Muscular and skeletal issues are also increasingly common, affecting almost all adults over 30, whether or not they are aware of it yet.*

- *Those few adults and children who play regular sport offset some of the automatic damage that a sedentary existence supplies. Most sports come with serious drawbacks however, and few sports can be relied on for a Total Fitness Programme.*

References:

1. NHS (2011) Statistics on Obesity, Physical Activity and Diet in England [Online] Available at: http://www.ic.nhs. uk/webfiles/publications/003_Health_Lifestyles/opad11/Statistics_on_Obesity_Physical_Activity_and_Diet_ England_2011_revised_Aug11.pdf

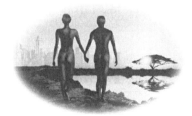

CHAPTER FOUR

Don't Take Your Health Advice from Your Government, Doctor, Family or Friends

"If you tell a lie big enough and keep repeating it, people will eventually come to believe it"

Joseph Goebbels
(Reich Minister of Public Enlightenment and Propaganda)

Some things in life we just have to take on faith – because, after all, life is too short. Is Andrex softer than other loo papers? Who knows? Who cares? However, there are other things – such as your health, your body, your wellness and ultimately your happiness – that if you choose to take on unquestioning trust could result in a life that's just *too* short."

The subjects that this book addresses should not be left to blind faith.

It's all too easy for us to believe that science now has all the answers. When you see how much we have learnt over the centuries, it's easy to believe that we are now close to knowing most of what needs to be known. The thing is that people have *always* felt like this at every stage of science's development. Within the last hundred years or so, some of the world's best scientists have believed the following:

- *That only a continually expanding earth can explain earthquakes and mountain ranges.*
- *That phrenology (the study of the size and shape of individuals' heads) can show their personality.*
- *That electric shock therapy and lobotomies are humane and effective treatments for depression and mental disorders.*

Ideas like this were, until recently, taken as gospel but, with the gift of hindsight, we can see just how many 19th and 20th century 'facts' were actually nothing but folly.

Even when science or new learning disproves commonly held notions, it often takes *decades* for the facts to permeate into the consciousness of ordinary people.

Recognise these facts?

- *Vikings wore horns on their helmets*
- *The Great Wall of China is the only man-made object that can be seen from space*
- *Bats are blind and rely on sonar*
- *Goldfish have short memories*

Not facts at all – sorry! All the evidence suggests that all these ideas are totally untrue - no matter how deep these beliefs have been drilled into our minds. However it'll probably be at least another 5-10 years before the *new* facts and the *new* evidence reach ordinary people who don't subscribe to New Scientist magazine.

We need to remember that many of the facts we were supplied with by teachers, scientists, parents, and textbooks will be overturned in the centuries to come and looked upon as curious remnants of an ill-informed past. Many of today's truths are tomorrow's quaintly-recalled superstitions.

Is it just possible that in the world of nutrition (a fledgling subject at best), we have got some things terribly wrong and inside-out?

For me at least, entertaining that possibility has allowed me to obtain results for myself and my clients that I rarely see elsewhere. All I urge is this:

Keep An Open Mind!

I am not asking you to trust me. Despite my experience of seeing the right results time after time with my clients, and my unrelenting passion for expanding my knowledge of and perfecting my approach to this topic, I don't want you to simply take my word for anything.

I *will* however, ask you to *trust yourself*. I urge you to make up your own mind about things. In the end that's all any of us can do. Certainly, while you should lend weight to what supposedly qualified individuals tell you, it's up to *you* to decide what makes sense.

> *"Trust your own instinct. Your mistakes might as well be*
> *your own, instead of someone else's."*
>
> **Billy Wilder**

This is the key thing about Instinctive Fitness. I am not a self-proclaimed expert (of which we have enough already) telling you that you *must* do this or *must* do that. I am not setting myself up as an all-knowing guru or pretending that I have all the answers. I'm certainly not pretending that I know *all* the science. (I would be suspicious of anyone who makes this claim.) All I can do is tell you *what* I do and *why* I do it. The results I get – both for me and my clients – speak for themselves. This whole book was written to urge you to become an explorer; a pioneer in one of the last uncharted territories for many human beings: the land of self.

The title of this book urges you to honour and defend your *instincts* – your own instinct for what holds good and true *for you*. Then, by paying attention to the feedback your own body offers, you can decide for yourself whether any particular idea is worth its salt. Listening closely to this feedback is essential because we are not all identical. That's why a one-size-fits-all approach will never get the best results.

If you notice, for example, that you feel tired every time you eat bananas (even though I might have said that fruit is healthy and natural) then stop eating them! If coffee upsets your digestion then it's got to go! If you are exhausted when exercising five days a week, then you're doing too much, too hard – no matter what anybody tells you. You must find your own way through the modern maze of life, not rely too heavily on someone else's map. It's about getting to know your true self, free on any of the conditioning with which we have all been brought up.

Any logic, rhetoric or studies employed in this book really aren't another attempt to give you an alternative brain-washing. They are there simply to create enough doubt about what we're all been told – and convince you to try something different instead.

I would urge you to listen to as many sides of the argument as you can, then think about the issue yourself and reach workable conclusions that you can apply to your own life. Many of the ideas I'm going to put forward aren't just hypothetical: **they are easily testable.**

A little challenge to you…your first fitness experiment.

If I tell you that pushing yourself hard on the treadmill for 30 minutes four times a week isn't a good way to lose weight, then try it! Ensure you control other variables – don't suddenly start a strict starvation diet at the same time for example – and see how you fare over 4 weeks. If you don't get much weight loss (which is my prediction), try slowing down to a walk for 30 minutes three times a week and adding 5 minutes of uphill interval sprints at the end. For best results try it in the morning without taking breakfast. See if that works. (I say it will, but what does it matter to you what I think?)

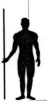

What did our ancestors do?

I'll now suggest that the above *will* work for you because, as humans, we evolved to do plenty of walking in a day, with maybe a little jogging and infrequent bursts of speed. We did not evolve to be regular marathon racers. The ability to cover long distances as fast as possible was not a useful function when most daily movement involved the need to judicially stalk animals or forage for food with all our senses finely attuned to our environment. Crashing around at high speed would give our position away to prey and cause us to pass by any useful flora or fauna without noticing its presence.

If the above makes sense to you, I think you'll be well motivated to take this little piece of weight loss advice. If you disagree, you might dismiss it. Or you might try it anyway, just to prove I'm wrong.

In the Middle Ages, everybody 'knew' that black cats were a source of bad luck: it was common knowledge. Your local minister would also have been able to tell you definitively that the earth was a few thousand years old and flat. What are we being misled about on health today?

Question Everything ('No, why should I?')

What really matters is that you don't just take anybody's prescription for health (or politics, ethics, religion, or whatever) at face value because of the perceived 'authority' of the source or because of how widely a belief is held.

The prevalence of a belief in no way indicates its validity.

Remember that the first trick of majority opinion in defending its position is to turn something that is nothing more than a shared *belief* into something that appears to the unwary as an undisputed *fact*. The second trick is then to close ranks and ridicule any conflicting ideas that challenge that group's accepted standing.

However, despite a tick-box education system designed to fill us with the knowledge we 'need', rather than to empower us to actually *think* for ourselves, there have always been people who are unafraid to challenge accepted orthodoxies. There have always been people willing to question the laziness, fear, apathy or self-interest of the majority - and it is these people who change the world!

"Thus to be independent of public opinion is the first formal condition of achieving anything great"

G.W.F. Hegel

I simply urge you to be one of these questioning people – at the very least challenging the things that really matter to you. I hope you'll agree with me that the longevity and quality of the rest of your life should definitely fall into that category.

Is this a conspiracy or just plain incompetence?

The establishment has spent millions of pounds telling us how we should live our lives in order to enjoy good health, pumping out fact after fact to supposedly reduce the strain of a health service buckling under the weight of citizens who live so long, but are unwell for much of it.

For the last 20 years or so, the British Government and its Department of Health – neither of which trust you to think for yourself – have generally been singing the same sort of tune, whilst quietly changing some very important lyrics. We have been told repeatedly, for example, that in order to control our weight and minimise the chance of cardiovascular disease we should eat a **"low-fat diet"** and enjoy **"healthy grains and vegetables"**.

While this message hasn't really changed for some time, we have been warned off certain foods like butter, lard, red meat and full-fat milk – and even, at one time, eggs![1] The establishment is still firmly of the position that the higher levels of saturated fat found in these products are damaging to health.

On the back of these largely unsubstantiated claims – claims which the British public have gobbled up greedily – other products have appeared to replace these allegedly dangerous products. Examples of these are margarine (which has been around since the last world war but has grown massively in popularity over recent decades), skimmed and homogenised milk, highly-processed vegetable oils, artificial sweeteners and a huge number of instant processed meals.

In general, the British people have taken this anti-fat message to heart and have bought anything in sight with the words 'low-fat' printed on them. In fact we now eat less fat than we have ever done, and we take in most of our calories in the form of breads, pastas, biscuits, pastries, rice and potatoes. The majority of these products are made from grain (potatoes being the exception), and particularly wheat. What all of these products have in common is that they are massively **high-carbohydrate products**.

Carbohydrates are foods that the body burns by converting it into **glucose**, which is just a form of sugar, and it converts that into *glycogen* which is stored in the liver and muscles ready to be deployed as energy.

The sugar paradox

The other part of the low-fat message endorsed by our government and health gurus is that we also need to avoid **sugar** if we hope to improve our health and lose weight. Products like Coke, ice-cream and sweets are criticised for the high levels of sugar they contain (and rightly so).

Have you noticed the big contradiction in this line of thinking? It should be quite easy to spot from looking at the last few paragraphs. If we get most of our calories from carbohydrates instead of fat, and carbs break down into sugar, then we're going to be eating *an awful lot of sugar* whether we intend to or not. This is the very same sort of sugar that we are told, in the next piece of the confusing puzzle, we should avoid.

Now the above is of course a simplified description of the very complicated chemical reactions that go on in the body. I don't want to give the impression that there's nothing more to it than this, but nor do I want to offer a first year course in Bio-Chemistry.

However, in essence, the case goes like this: **in order to avoid the fat which we are told is bad for us, we are told to eat plenty of carbohydrates. Carbohydrates quickly turn into sugar, a substance we are told by the exact same sources is bad for us!** Sugar, if not burned through exercise, encourages the body to store fat. It also disrupts our blood-sugar levels and, in the longer term, moves us steadily in the direction of diabetes. Go figure, as the Americans are fond of saying.

You might wonder if this apparent 'Catch 22' is unavoidable though. Perhaps there is no alternative but to turn to this carb-heavy diet if fat is so bad for us; but that's a big 'if', so we'd better examine the evidence for this claim against fat.

Baffled and bamboozled by science?

The 'Seven Countries Study', started in the 1950s by Ancel Keys, provided doctors and scientists with enough authority to change the way we would eat for the next four decades. Key's study looked at the correlation between saturated fat and heart disease across 22 different countries.

The published results, however, included data from only the 7 of the 22 countries that he studied that showed some sort of link. The other 15 countries were excluded from the study because the data collected did not support the hypothesis that Keys was tasked to find.

Although Keys' study really wasn't very honest science[2], commentators and the medical establishment claimed that his results showed that an increased intake of saturated fat was directly linked to an increased incidence of cardiovascular disease. However, amongst the data he deliberately omitted (15 countries' worth!) was evidence that showed the direct opposite of the link for which he was looking. That data included the diets of the Masai (with a diet dominated by red meat, milk and blood), the Inuit who we've already discussed (who just eat high-blubber animals) and the Tokelau (who get more than 50% of their calories from saturated fat). All of these groups eat massive quantities of saturated fat and suffer from almost no cardio-vascular disease whatsoever.[3]

When the data from all 22 countries was considered there was almost no correlation between these factors at all.

It certainly can't be denied that saturated fats are sometimes found in the diet of those people with cardiovascular difficulties, but it doesn't follow from this that saturated fats *cause* heart disease.

In Ancel Keys' study, selective data was used to suggest that a link existed, whereas, in point of fact, when all the data is considered, there wasn't one. However, that wasn't what he was being *paid* to find.

Right now, even in 2012, studies are still being churned out to order, scare-mongering about the consumption of red meat. However they still fail to account properly for differences between processed meat and natural meat, and between intensive industrial farming (with its reliance on antibiotics and steroids) and meat provided by from properly fed, pastured animals.

As you know, any good scientific study should change only one variable at a time to isolate the exact variable which caused the change in results. However, follow-up studies of population groups suggested that those eating more red meat (a source of saturated fat) are more prone to disease, but failed to note that these people were also those eating the most processed food, the most processed meat, the most junk food, the most salt, and the most sugar.

As a result of unscientific and insecure studies like these, the British people are now told to eat no more than two portions of red meat a week, to avoid butter, and to choose skimmed milk, margarine and vegetable oils. When the press use phrases like 'artery-clogging saturated fat' it's easy to see how a natural substance – our body's primary fuel source and a substance that much of our body is composed of – has become so demonised.

This is normally where someone says "but saturated fat causes cholesterol deposits in the arteries, and excess high cholesterol can cause heart-attacks."

I'll deal with this in depth in Chapter Six, but suffice to say here that the production of cholesterol seems to be perhaps the most maligned natural process that our body performs. Here again, cause and effect have been placed the wrong way around. The facts suggest that excess cholesterol[4] does not actually cause harm to the body at all, but is in actual fact the body's attempt to *heal* itself. Instead, damage to the body (in the form of inflammation and oxidation) cause the body to patch up the damage with the intelligent use of cholesterol.

To think otherwise is like believing that sticky plasters cause cuts because they are often found together in the same place.

Too often in science, correlation is mistaken for causation. For example:

Seagulls are often found following fishing trawlers around, so we can tell that trawlers cause the production of seagulls.

(…or perhaps it's the seagulls causing fishing trawlers?)

Both are ridiculous of course; we can understand this on a common sense level; all these factors just occur together because of a third, unconsidered variable – in this case, of course, their common presence is explained by a mutual interest in fish. However, we don't generally have the knowledge to spot the same error in specialist areas when promulgated by 'experts'.

It would seem bizarre if what was our main food source for the vast majority of our evolutionary history (red meat with its 'dangerous' cholesterol and 'artery clogging' fat) is actually a danger to our health. If this is true, it makes me wonder how human beings ever survived as a species at all. We might as well suggest that grass is bad for cows or that primates should avoid fruit.

Actually, if the results of all subsequent studies are viewed not through the lens of one originally flawed theory, but through the open eyes of objectivity, the reverse seems nearer to the truth: there is in fact plenty of evidence that actually demonstrates the *benefits* of increased fat and cholesterol in our diets.

Naughty fat munching countries

Between 1958 and 1999, the **Japanese** doubled their protein intake, ate 400 per cent more fat and their cholesterol levels went up by 20 per cent. If Keys was right, they should have dropped like flies – but did they? No. Their stroke rate, which had been the highest in the world, was reduced seven fold, while deaths from heart attacks dropped by 50 per cent.

Then there's the **French**. They eat much more saturated fat than we do in Britain; they smoke more, take less exercise, and have the same cholesterol levels; they also have the same average blood pressure. However, ignoring Paris (which no longer consumes a traditional diet), the French have considerably lower rates of obesity and *one quarter* of the rate of heart disease that we do. This fact has confused (and is more often ignored by) so many scientists that it's become known as the French Paradox.

Numerous surveys of traditional populations have yielded statistics that confound all those who have sought to indoctrinate us in the dangers of saturated fat. For example, a study comparing Jews living in **Yemen**, whose diets contained fats only of an animal origin, to Yemenite Jews living in Israel, whose diets contained margarine and vegetable oils, showed little heart disease or diabetes in the former group but high levels of both diseases in the latter.[5]

A comparison of populations in northern and southern India revealed a similar pattern. People in northern **India** consume 17 times more animal fat but have an incidence of coronary heart disease seven times lower than people in southern India.[6]

The **Masai** and kindred tribes of Africa subsist largely on beef, blood and milk (they drink the blood of their cattle). However they are largely free from coronary heart disease and have excellent blood cholesterol levels.[7]

The **Inuit** eat inordinately large quantities of animal fats from fish and sea animals. Those who still eat the traditional diet are free of disease and exceptionally hardy.[8]

This isn't a case of 'the exception proves the rule'; there are many more examples of countries confounding the prejudices of the low-fat propaganda wagon. Follow this footnote for more.[9] And anyway...

How can ancient foods cause a modern disease?
Does that make any sense?

Actually, posed more accurately, the question is: **How can ancient foods that we eat in lower quantities than ever before, be causing modern diseases that we almost never had in the past?**

You only have to look back to the 1930s to find a time when people were eating large amounts of saturated fat in the UK. Even though 'healthy' margarine made from seed-oils hadn't been introduced as a replacement for 'dangerous' butter and lard, there were almost no cases of heart disease or lung cancer, despite the fact that 80% of the population smoked!

However, on the back of Keys' highly dubious study, a whole new approach to dieting was formed and food companies rushed to produce new foods to fulfil the demand for 'healthy', low-fat products and to fill their own coffers. We will look at these some more in Chapter Eight when we consider 'Real Food'.

The sad fact is that there was a need for a study showing *fat equals heart attack* and, although the results of Keys' study didn't really show that at all, it was enough for the author to appear on the front page of 'Time Magazine' and a whole new, low-fat approach to health was born. The *theory* that saturated fat was unhealthy was hammered into our consciousness by foul play:

'The Lipid Hypothesis' was promoted to Lipid Fact!

Since that time, in the UK and the USA we have run a fifty year experiment into the effects of this baseless leap into the dark. The findings aren't pretty, as we found in the last chapter, but too many people in power have a vested interest in the status quo to change tack.

As the population of the UK and beyond continue to cut healthy fats from their diets, I'm reminded of Einstein's definition of insanity as "continuing to do the same thing but expecting a different result."

In this chapter I hope I have shown how successive governments have inadvertently collaborated out of sheer desperation with both the medical industry and the self-interest of the processed food industry. In doing so, they have effectively told us what to think and closed our minds to considering other possibilities, even when it is only too apparent to those who dare look that this mass-engineered experiment has not worked. The end result is that the whole way we think about health and weight loss has become tainted.

The truth finally wakes from its slumber

There have, of course, been other opinions expressed over the years which have been systematically shouted down to save face and maintain the status quo. However, these voices are now becoming increasingly more numerous, and are at last starting to be heard.

The largest of these is the **low-carb movement** which has grown over the last 10 years to become the biggest thorn in the side of 'conventional wisdom'. This new movement has gathered followers through the medium of the internet and huge quantities of positive anecdotal testimonials. More recently, meta-studies (studies of studies) of diets have also shown 'low-carb diets' to be more successful than 'low-fat' as a weight-loss approach.[10]

At last, it seems that although the establishment is not yet ready to listen, we as the population are crying out to try something different. And this means, for the moment, ignoring the official line that stubbornly refuses to change – despite being ridiculed daily by the ever-growing statistics that prove its abject failure.

Key Chapter points

● *Listen to advice, but decide for yourself on matters of importance. Logic is better than blind faith, but self-experimentation can be the ultimate litmus test.*

● *Bad science and a desperate establishment have brainwashed us to fear fat. Fat is your friend. You're made of the stuff - it's supposed to be your principal fuel.*

● *The 'low-fat and healthy grains' ideology has failed us. Look around you.*

● *You can't trust the food industry to feed you well. They care about their profit, not your health.*

● *You can't trust the government either; it's in the thrall of the big food giants and their manipulative lobby groups.*

● *Low-carb is the future, but don't wait to be told 'officially'! The establishment hates u-turns!*

All diets, apart from the one endorsed by 2.5 million years of evolution, are based on fads not facts.

References:

1. Recently however, the government health warning on eggs has been rescinded (read: U-turn). Fears about eggs raising cholesterol levels were acknowledged to be erroneous now that it has been accepted that eggs are only high in one particular sort of cholesterol, one that they now concede isn't harmful. The other, they're still not happy about.

2. Wikipedia (2012) Uffe Ravnskov [Online] Available at: http://en.wikipedia.org/wiki/Uffe_Ravnskov#Investigation_of_the_Lipid_Hypothesis.2C_or_.22Diet-Heart.22_Idea

3. Ho K-J et al. (1971) "Studies on the Masai." Archeological Pathology, 91:387; Mann GV, et al. (1972) "Atherosclerosis in the Maasai." American Journal of Epidemiology, 95:26-37

4. Pinckney ER, Pinckney C (1973) The Cholesterol Controversy, Sherbourne Press, Los Angeles

5. Cohen A (1963) "Fats and carbohydrates as factors in atheroclerosis and diabetes in Yemenite Jews." Am Heart J, 65:291

6. Malhotra, S, (1968) Indian Journal of Industrial Medicine, 14:219

7. Ho K-J et al. (1971) "Studies on the Masai." Archeological Pathology, 91:387; Mann GV, et al. (1972) "Atherosclerosis in the Maasai." American Journal of Epidemiology, 95:26-37

8. Price, W (1945) DDS, Nutrition and Physical Degeneration, Price-Pottenger Nutrition Foundation, San Diego, CA, 59-72.

9. Several Mediterranean societies have low rates of heart disease even though fat —including highly saturated fat from lamb, sausage and goat cheese—comprises up to 70% of their caloric intake. The inhabitants of Crete, for example, are remarkable for their good health and longevity. Willett WC et al. (1995) "Mediterranean diet pyramid: a cultural model for healthy eating" Am J Clin Nutr, June 1995, 61:1402S - 1406S; Perez-Llamas F et al (1996) "Estimates of food intake and dietary habits in a random sample of adolescents in south-east Spain" J Hum Nutr Diet, Dec 1996, 9:6:463-471; Alberti-Fidanza, A, et al, Eur J Clin Nutr, Feb 1994, 48:2:85-91

A study of Puerto Ricans revealed that, although they consume large amounts of animal fat, they have a very low incidence of colon and breast cancer. Fernandez NA (1975) "Nutrition in Puerto Rico" Cancer Res, 35:3272-3291; Martines I et al. (1975) "Cancer Incidence in the United States and Puerto Rico" Cancer Res, 35:3265 -3271.

A study of the long-lived inhabitants of Soviet Georgia revealed that those who eat the most fatty meat live the longest. Pitskhelauri GZ (1982) The Long Living of Soviet Georgia, Human Sciences Press, New York, NY

In Okinawa, where the average life span for women is 84 years—longer than in Japan—the inhabitants eat generous amounts of pork and seafood and do all their cooking in lard. The Swiss live almost as long on one of the fattiest diets in the world. Tied for third in the longevity stakes are Austria and Greece—both with high-fat diets. Moore TJ (1990) Lifespan: What Really Affects Human Longevity, Simon and Schuster, New York, NY. None of these studies is mentioned by those urging restriction of saturated fats.

Other than Keys, the 'Framingham Study' is always cited as the 'evidence' for the flawed Lipid Hypothesis. However, after 40 years, the director stated: "The more saturated fat one ate, the more cholesterol one ate, the more calories one ate, the lower the person's serum cholesterol...we found that the people who ate the most cholesterol, ate the most saturated fat, ate the most calories, weighed the least and were the most physically active."

10. Hession M et al. (2008) "Systematic review of randomized controlled trials of low-carbohydrate vs. low-fat/low-calorie diets in the management of obesity and its comorbidities". Obesity Reviews 10(1): 36-50.

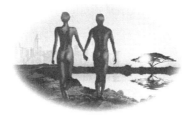

CHAPTER FIVE

A Fork in the Road

"Every human being has a two million year old man within himself; if he loses contact with that two million year old self, he loses his real roots"

Laurens Van de Post

In this chapter I am going to give you some historical perspective. Once you see where we now stand, I think you'll have a clearer idea about how to move forward. As we begin to understand the problem more thoroughly, the answers will begin to emerge.

You'll learn how it can be that we've got quite so far off track, so quickly. You'll understand why it is that, unlike other members of the animal kingdom, few of us can still trust our natural instincts any more when it comes to staying fit and well.

Let's go right, right back: back to the time when human-like species first walked out of the African forest on two legs. They did this because they no longer needed to spend all their time in the trees and, after thousands of years, had evolved to the point where they were more comfortable looking for food on the ground than they were climbing about for it in the canopy. For the first time, humans stayed on the savannah and began to look around for new food sources which would mean they wouldn't have to depend on tree-borne fruit in the way that their semi-human ancestors had.

Their natural foods became the animals, nuts, berries, roots, fruits and vegetables that they found around them. There was usually an abundant supply of food with natural seasonal variation. In time they learnt how to fish and, later, how to cook.

Cooking was a crucial evolutionary step, as it meant that calories could be digested more easily. Food could be eaten more quickly and less energy was used digesting food as it was already partly completed by the cooking process. This meant good access to the vitamins and minerals they needed, loads of calories, and lots of spare time.

This spare time and improved nutrition meant that over thousands of years our ancestors grew in stature, knowledge, language skills and development. More of their time was used for play, artistic endeavour, weapon making, and socialisation.

Greater intelligence raises a human being's chances of survival and procreation so, over the course of many millennia, an evolutionary slide towards being a species with superior intelligence was the natural result.

For the next million years or so, humans continued to grow as a species. Mankind became bigger, cleverer, more sophisticated creatures, capable of adapting to a growing number of different habitats. They studied their environment and learnt new behaviours to cope with new challenges. Those that were incapable of such changes did not survive long enough to pass on their weaker genes through their progeny.

There grew a mass of accumulated wisdom that each tribe possessed and passed onto the next generation through tribal wisdom, example, tradition and rite. Each new generation was taught by the older one where to fish, how to hunt, where to find edible fungi, how to build shelters; all the things needed to live life off the land.

During this time, and for most of their existence, they were nomadic or semi-nomadic. If they had 'homes' they were temporary structures or natural dwelling places (like caves). It was essential for them to be able to remain mobile. When the game, flora or fauna in an area became too poor, they needed to be able to move on. They may also have followed the path of migrating animals (antelope for example) and changed area according to the season. There was no obvious reason to stay in one place for very long.

All of this changed with the advent of farming. With the discovery of grain and the milling process, for the very first time, humans had an almost guaranteed source of calories. (I say almost: crops *do* fail!) This meant that the possibility of starvation was considerably lowered... or at least appeared to be. The ability to produce food in greater quantities also supported a growing population and larger families.

The trade-off for this new way of life was considerable. So great, in fact, that some thinkers consider the advent of agriculture to be the greatest mistake our race has ever made. Professor Jared Diamond makes a brilliant case for this in his book "Guns, Germs and Steel".[1]

Men gave up their hunter status and became workers of the land. They had to work long hours and spend much time physically grinding grain with basic pestle and mortar equipment. Women also gave up their role as foragers in favour of rearing more children and supporting their partners on farms or small-holdings. More time also had to be put aside for the preparation and cooking of these new grains.

The discovery of farming meant that previously inedible foods could now be consumed. Crops such as barley, wheat and rye could not have been eaten before because, as wild cereals, they had their own defences that prevented most animals from ingesting them; these plants contain large quantities of toxins which mean that animals are forced to leave them alone and search for more edible alternatives. The new milling process meant that, with lots of work, these plants could now be digested by human beings and fed to their cattle. This changed everything.

Humans changed from food sources that were entirely edible – and that they had adapted to eating over millions of years – to a new grain-based diet which was more dependable, but only partially digestible. Toxins which had originally prevented its consumption were still present in the grain, but in smaller quantities that posed less immediate danger. As well as containing these toxins, these foods also lacked the nutritional value of the foods they replaced.

Cumulatively, the adoption of these grains as the mainstay of a human diet lowered the health of our species. Within a small amount of time, humans developed a new range of diseases, grew shorter in stature and became dependent on farmed land for their survival.

These effects are well documented in the relatively recent science of Paleopathology, which is the study of signs of disease in ancient people. Scientists in this field are able to identify the moment the switch to agriculture took place in various parts of the world with surprising accuracy. They do this by examining Paleolithic rubbish dumps where ancient excrement reveals the switch from wild plants and animals to cultivated crops.

They can subsequently compare the food eaten with what the skeletons or the preserved bodies of these humans can tell us. Sometimes we can learn as much from a well-preserved corpse as a modern pathologist can tell from a recently deceased one.

A skeleton reveals more than its owner's sex, weight, and approximate age. In cases where there are many skeletons, the expected life span and risk of death at any given age can be calculated. Paleopathologists can work out growth rates by measuring the bones of people of different ages, examining teeth for enamel defects (signs of childhood malnutrition), and recognising scars left on bones by anaemia, tuberculosis, leprosy, and other diseases.

One measurable factor that tells us a lot about the health of a given race of people is height. Skeletons from Greece and Turkey show that the average height of early hunter-gatherers was 5' 9" for men and 5' 5" for women. With the arrival of agriculture, heights fell; by 3000 B.C. they had reached a low of only 5' 3" for men and 5 foot for women. Modern Greeks and Turks have still not regained the average height of their distant ancestors.

Another good example is seen in the work of George Armelagos and his colleagues working at the University of Massachusetts.[2] They found 800 skeletons in burial mounds in the Illinois and Ohio River valleys which showed that these early farmers paid a price when they moved to the intensive farming of maize. Compared to the hunter-gatherers who preceded them, these farmers had a nearly 50 per cent increase in enamel defects (indicative of malnutrition); a four-fold increase in iron-deficiency anaemia; a three-fold increase in bone lesions, reflecting infectious disease; and an increase in degenerative conditions of the spine, probably reflecting a lot of hard, repetitive physical labour.

The main reason for these findings is that while hunter-gatherers enjoyed a varied diet, **early farmers obtained most of their food from just a few starchy crops.** The farmers gained cheap calories at the cost of poor nutrition. They concentrated their efforts on producing high-yield, high-carbohydrate crops like rice and potatoes, whereas the mix of wild plants and animals in the diets of surviving hunter-gatherers provided more protein and essential fatty acids, and gave a better balance of other nutrients.

Today, just three high-carbohydrate plants – wheat, rice, and corn – provide the bulk of the calories consumed by the human species, yet each one is deficient in vitamins and amino acids essential to life. In the 21st century, we eat a more varied diet than these early farmers, but these high-carbohydrate plants still represent the majority of our calories.

Another reason for the findings is that these farmers were forced to work much harder than hunter-gatherers to survive. They would perform manual labour (which you might think would keep them fit) but without sufficient recovery time meaning that, like the marathon runners we mentioned earlier, the toll on their health was great.

For comparison, we have a good idea of how hard our hunter-gatherer ancestors worked because scattered across the world there are several dozen groups of so-called primitive people, like the Kalahari Bushmen or the Hadza of Tanzania, who continue to support themselves in a way that has remained unchanged throughout history. These people have plenty of leisure time, sleep a good deal, and work less hard than their farming neighbours. For instance, the average time devoted to obtaining food is only 12 to 19 hours a week for the Bushmen, while the nomadic Hadza work for less than 14 hours.

Early farmers, by contrast, worked most or all of the daylight hours and possibly after dark too, by candlelight.

You might expect that eventually humans would evolve to cope with this new way of living, and this new, partially-toxic food matter. However, for evolution to change anything it has to change the propensity for an animal to die *before* it can pass on its genes to its offspring. Farming didn't do this.

In fact, farming ensured that many of the natural dangers that befell semi-nomadic man were removed from the range of possible early deaths. They were also less likely to die early as a result of starvation. Less genetically-gifted human beings were now able to survive and pass their genes onto a new generation. This was effectively the end of large-scale evolutionary improvement for the human race as selection pressure was completely removed from the population. (The idea that our DNA today is identical to that of our primal ancestors is supported by hundreds of leading anthropologists, evolutionary biologists and genetic researchers[3]).

Instead, farming meant that most adults were able to stay alive long enough to procreate and then, maybe 10 years later, in their 30s, would die of one of the many diseases that attacked their weakened immune systems and prematurely-aged bodies. In this way, no evolutionary preference for 'good digesters of grains' could ever be established.

Many more people were now surviving, but they were doing no more than struggling through a growing list of ailments to what we would call early middle age. They would have been lucky to see their children reach the end of their teens.

It's important to remember that, in evolutionary terms, this trend towards grain cultivation is a flash in the pan. If the history of the human race, to put it on a simple scale, began at midnight, and we've just finished our first day on the earth, then only in last *four seconds* have we stopped being hunter-gatherers in favour of mass-produced agriculture. However obvious a fuel source grain might seem to us in the 21st century, it has only been a consumable option for a tiny fraction of our time on this planet.

The evidence seems to suggest that we are paying a very dear price for these last few seconds!

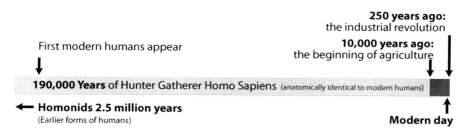

250 years ago:
the industrial revolution

First modern humans appear

10,000 years ago:
the beginning of agriculture

190,000 Years of Hunter Gatherer Homo Sapiens (anatomically identical to modern humans)

← **Homonids 2.5 million years**
(Earlier forms of humans)

Modern day

Another key, but arguably less dramatic moment was the arrival of the **Industrial Revolution**. Many people were freed from the need to work on small farms in the production of food. Instead, the century of the **factory** was upon us. Men, women and children looked to factories to survive. Ignoring the titled aristocracy, there were two types of people: those who owned factories and those who worked in them. The huge majority fell into the second camp.

Conditions in factories were so grim (as they still are in much of the third world) that a life toiling in the fields in the sunlight and in contact with nature could only be regarded as a rustic idyll. Painters and poets of the Romantic period depicted idealised scenes of country folk living simple but worthy lives, while their city-bound cousins were as cooped up and maltreated as a modern battery hen. Cramped conditions and overcrowding led to stress, disease and further malnutrition.

Only with the most recent of our revolutions have we been saved from the miserable fate that befell the common man. The **Technological Revolution** meant that factories became automated and a majority of people were paid for their ability to provide a service, communicate, create or teach. All of this can be done without the concentrated manual labour that had been a feature of working lives in the past.

At the same time, our domestic lives have also changed forever. We no long need to wash our clothes by hand or walk to the shops; no firewood needs collecting; the lawn can be mown by a petrol-driven machine and the tree in the garden can be taken down with a chainsaw.

With new technology we no longer needed to use our bodies for most common household tasks. In fact we now need put in no more physical labour at home than we do in the work place.

Meanwhile, the complexity of our lives has increased. More technology means more opportunities, which mean more learning, which means more pressure – for both adults and children. Increasingly, schooling has had to become more intensive to ensure basic mastery of the complex skills we need to find a position in the workforce. This means that there is less time and fewer daylight hours available for children to run, jump and play as they have done for millennia. Added to this, a preference for entertainment based around technology (such as television, games consoles and mobile phones) means that even if they have the time, many children no longer have the inclination for physical play that they once did.

The Technological Revolution meant that, on-top of a high-calorie, high-carb diet, many of the modern generation live a lifestyle devoid of any physical endeavour at all. It also meant that new, heavily processed foods entered our diet in concentrations that our bodies have not evolved to cope with.

Here in the 21st century, all this has caught up with us. Clearly we can't just turn back the clock in some sort of revisionist, Luddite manner (though this might still happen if we run out of oil, as my dad likes to point out!) but there must be a better alternative to the path of madness we now tread.

Here is the problem as I see it:

We are human beings living in a radically different, modern world - but our unchanged stone-age genes expect the same challenges and environment that our ancient ancestors faced.

Our lives have changed, but our bodies and our natural instincts haven't evolved to keep up. We are Stone Age people living in the age of the

Microchip. This mismatch between gene and environment expresses itself in discomfort, disease, and compromised health and happiness.

What Darwin taught us:

The theory of evolution posits the idea that natural selection will favour those people (or, more accurately, *genes*; c.f "The Selfish Gene", Richard Dawkins, 1976) who possess traits that allow them to survive and breed where others will fail. In this way, human beings have adapted over millennia to their environment – psychologically, physiologically and genetically speaking – and have made a comfortable match.

Our ancestors evolved over millions of years under certain environmental conditions. These conditions (such as the foods they ate, the amount of sun they got, and the sort of movement that was required of them to survive, etcetera) shaped their genome. While the world has changed in innumerable ways, in the last 10,000 years (for better and worse), the human genome has changed very little and thus only thrives under similar conditions. Simply put, if you want a good future you had better look to your past.

Over the last few thousand years, our lifestyles have changed far more rapidly than evolution has been able to keep up with. The result of this is that humans are no longer perfectly adapted to their environment: backs hurt from sitting in chairs; eyes weaken from close reading all day; and waists fatten from little exercise and an abundance of cheap, empty calories.

Humans have changed their environment so quickly that although their high-tech lives appear much easier, there is a hidden price to pay in each deviation from the lifestyle we are genetically predisposed to expect.

I am not suggesting re-enacting cave-dwellers' lifestyles, so much as using their daily lives as a template to create a **logical framework** from which to produce an **optimal plan for health**. This means directing your gene expression toward longevity, wellness, fat burning and muscle building, and away from fat storing, muscle wasting, disease and illness. You'll start to learn how to do this in the next chapter.

Key Chapter Points

- *Evidence suggests that humans became shorter, weaker and less healthy when they abandoned the life of the hunter-gatherer to cultivate crops.*

- *The Industrial Revolution meant we could produce new crops on a huge scale. People had to work in the factories or fields for long hours.*

- *The Technological Revolution means that humans now have little reason to exert themselves or even move about much. A sedentary existence has ushered in a host of new problems.*

- *Little movement, when combined with a processed high-carb diet has partially crippled much of the western world. Our genes expect movement and real food.*

- *The government's attempts to help have often been hopelessly misplaced.*

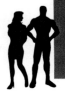

References

1. Diamond J (2005) Guns, Germs, and Steel: The Fates of Human Societies, WW Norton, New York.

2. Mummert A et al. (2011) "Stature and robusticity during the agricultural transition:Evidence from the bioarchaeological record." Economics and Human Biology 9:284-301.

3. For example, see the work of Dr. Boyd Eaton, chief anthropologist at Emory University in Atlanta and author of The Paleo Prescription and James V. Neel, of the University of Michigan's Department of Genetics

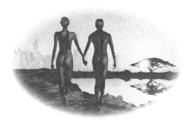

CHAPTER SIX

Natural Food

"Let food by thy medicine and medicine be thy food"

Hippocrates
(The Father of Modern Medicine)

"Eat Naturally Edible Food"

That's it. That's all I need to write in this chapter, but perhaps I should expand on that somewhat for those who consider a box of cereal a healthy option:

Don't eat: grains, sugar, starches, margarines, vegetable oils, or industrially-processed foods

There, it's said, point made; now you're ready to follow this great advice and discover that everything that you might hope for from a good eating plan is yours: low body-fat, good health, energy, optimal mood – everything.

What? You're not buying that? You say that your daily loaf is full of *whole grains* and your box of Frosted Flakes is *fortified with iron and minerals* so they must be good, right?

How could we all have been so misled?

This book isn't a science book and so it isn't aimed at anyone who has a penchant for wearing a lab coat. As in previous chapters I'm at pains not to switch off my intended reader, who probably isn't from a biochemical background. Here again I shall try my best to do the same, even at the risk that some will scream that I'm oversimplifying matters. I will try to ensure there is enough here to understand, to motivate, to take action on, and to get results from. I hope that is enough.

If you want a book that leans more heavily on science, I would point you in the direction of Gary Taubes's work, *"Good Calories, Bad Calories"*. Despite its slightly childish name, it's a monumental book outlining the difficulties we face with food choices in the modern world. Or try *"Why We Get Fat"* by the same author, which is also top science made as simple as possible.

I didn't want to write a science book that missed the people that this *really* matters to, so this chapter, like the others, is rather a book of concepts, ideas and the odd suggestion.

Here, put simply, is the situation and the problem as I see it:

As human beings, we evolved to eat anything around us that didn't present insurmountable toxic defences. In terms of foods this meant that we could eat animals (including seafood), most non-toxic insects (!), and non-toxic plants, seeds, nuts and roots.

Humans (in the form of homo sapiens) have been on the planet for the last 200,000 years. And for 190,000 of these we were big game hunters who consumed meat and plants in roughly equal measure.

Once the use of fire for cooking was discovered it became easier for us to consume more calories, because heating helps speed up the digestion of meats and plants. Raw food uses up a lot of calories just in its digestion.

These 100% natural freshly-killed prey, or straight-out-of-the-soil vegetation were the only foods we lived on for 190,000 years, right up until the agricultural revolution. At this point – going back only 5% of our time on the planet – some bright spark discovered a way of making a group of previously inedible foods – namely grains – *partially* edible.

Although we can never be 100% sure exactly what hunter-gathers ate (it must have varied from place to place anyway) **we do know what they didn't eat!**

Even a Whole Grain isn't a *Healthy* Grain!

Grains (as well as beans) could simply not be consumed by human beings until the advent of organised agriculture. Fossil records suggest that human health took a big hit with the advent of agriculture. We can tell from their bones that agriculturalists were shorter and had more cavities, smaller brains, and weaker bones than hunter-gatherers. Life expectancy also dropped dramatically.

Only around 100 years ago did food production become *fully* industrialised, leading to the appearance of vegetable oil, man-made trans-fats, cheap, fluffy white flour (originally produced specifically to prevent factory workers taking expensive toilet breaks), and inexpensive refined sugar. It also gave us a host of other new products which we allowed to be called foods. (It shouldn't come as news to you that, for example, jelly is not a real food, even though all of its constituent parts can be found in nature. It is a manufactured food – a product of food, not a food itself.)

The issue is this: no matter what we are lead to believe, most of these neological (new) foods are *still* partially toxic to human beings. Grains such as wheat, corn, barley and rye have allowed us to feed millions more people on our shrinking planet through the management of their growth. However, their presence in our diet has caused untold damage to our gut lining, to our immune systems, to our waist lines and to our health.[1]

Now I realise that if this is really the case, then this represents (as Al Gore might say) a seriously 'inconvenient truth', but there is a burgeoning number of nutritionists, researchers, scientists, and doctors who are coming around to this point of view. The Paleo Diet, upon which the Instinctive Fitness (IF) Programme leans heavily, eschews modern foods in favour of Paleolithic ones, and is one of the fastest growing dietary trends in the world. In the USA, it has gained a sizeable following as people abandon the failing advice of their government in favour of eating patterns that have been the foundation of every human being's development since before written history.

> **The proposition is this:** human beings have not evolved to eat processed high-carbohydrate foods, nor can they eat many modern, manufactured foods without long-term harm.

In Chapter Two I outlined the host of modern diseases to which humans have recently become more prone. With every passing year the list of diseases that revolve around the issue of increased inflammation and oxidisation of the organs and tissues grows more serious.

Whatever *is* doing this to us is rampant and out of control! So if at the end of this chapter you think that grain consumption and other modern toxins aren't the cause of all this misery, please let me know the better explanation you've come across. I beg you not to dismiss this chapter out of hand because of any short term 'inconvenience' its implications might cause you.

I would say that you at least owe it to yourself (and those who surround you) to try some of these ideas and see for yourself if they make a difference. I want to persuade you with logic initially, but ultimately I beg you to experiment with your own diet and find what works for *you*. Luckily, most people who make these changes are able to see and feel the changes reasonably quickly. There's just no need for blind faith.

> Why not give our 30 day challenge a try and see if you feel the difference yourself? Visit www.instinctive–fitness.com for our free 30 day workbook.

If you commit to making a few simple changes for just a few weeks with the 30-day challenge, I am confident that you *will* see enough of a difference to warrant sticking with the programme. Sure, it's not an overnight fix, but it will provide consistent workable results with a methodology you can stick to for the rest of your life. I assure you that the benefits will only continue to grow with passing time.

Are you ready for the 30-day challenge?

If you cut modern foods out of your life for at least a month, I guarantee you'll notice all or some of the following improvements:

- *Less addiction to food (though you'll still enjoy it)*
- *More consistent energy through the day*
- *No after-meal energy lag*
- *More resistance to cough, colds, flu, etc.*
- *Weight loss of at least 5 lbs (which will continue until you reach your ideal body weight)*
- *Clearer skin with fewer red patches and fewer allergic reactions*
- *A reduced waist-line (this sometimes happens independently of weight loss)*
- *An ability to miss meals without a feeling of weakness or desperation*
- *Less dependence on stimulants like coffee to stay awake and to maintain your mood*

Why does no-one else tell us this?

Because cutting grains out of your diet is bad for big industry? Consider not just the loss of sales in terms of grain itself, but also all the other industries making money out of patching up the ailments caused by grains!

Before you decide to accept or decline my 30-day challenge, I'd like to outline why I believe that taking these steps is the ONLY acceptable approach to improved health.

The first reason is simple – **all other diets are to a greater or lesser extent a fad**. Think about it, in terms of the millennia we've been on this small blue spinning planet – *everybody* in the western world is on a fad diet of one kind or another, Even if you just eat 'whatever', or the 'standard' British diet, or just whatever your partner puts in the fridge, you are still partaking in an entirely new experiment. All diets based around modern food are, through the long-seeing eyes of history, faddish; they are a flash in the pan in evolutionary terms.

And look at the decline in our health over the last 100 or so years we've been on this western diet 'fad.'

The diet of those in the 'developed' west

The diet that most of us eat now is fairly easy to describe. It is broadly similar to the one the British Government advises us to eat. That is to say, 'a balanced diet based around healthy grains, vegetables, and low in fat.' And that's where it all goes wrong.

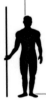

> The western diet is dominated by over-processed, high-carb, high-sugar, packaged 'bait food' peddled by the big corporations. It is food that is in fact designed specifically to hook you by your poor confused instincts straight to the checkout counter!

Here in Britain, **wheat** is the crop of choice (other countries have other poisons). Wheat is found in every bread, every cereal and every pasta. It's relatively cheap and we consume it by the skip-load. Of all the grains (like rye, barley and corn) wheat is the most abundant *and* the most harmful. In fact, half the people I know have a wheat-based cereal for breakfast, a sandwich for lunch, and often pasta for supper, meaning that they inadvertently take the majority of their calories from just this one harmful grain.

It's an undisputed medical fact that some people are unable to consume any bread, or anything made of most grains, because of the presence of **gluten**. Gluten is a protein molecule found in abundance in wheat. You'll have seen a growing number of gluten-free products in the shops which allow the celiac sufferer who cannot handle gluten to eat the same sort of products with *apparent* impunity.

However the obvious symptoms that celiac sufferers suffer from when they consume gluten are just the visible tip of a much bigger iceberg. They are just the small part of society who manifest *immediate* and *obvious* symptoms. The rest of us still suffer the effects too - just on a time delay of years rather than hours, building up problems over the course of a lifetime.

It's not just the *gluten* in the wheat either; it is the *rest* of the product that causes the problems. Wheat, like all grains, contains its own defence mechanisms. Unlike a grass which 'wishes' to be eaten by animals to disperse its seeds, a grain 'wishes' to repel animals from consuming it. To do so, it produces anti-nutrients such as ***gluten, lectins*** and ***phytates,*** which actually damage the reproductive tracts of any animal that tries to eat it. That, of course, is the reason that these plants remained untouched by us for so many millennia.

> Then, 10,000 years ago, some genius came up with a cunning way to grow, harvest and mill these grains to make them consumable, and they thought they were onto a winner. They discovered that some of these defensive toxins could be removed through an easy process.

A very modern fluffy, white loaf

One of the main problems with this sort of high-carb fare is that our modern breads are baked to be light and fluffy, and they are almost all universally awful in their ingredients. There isn't really much difference, nutritionally-speaking, between white and brown bread, despite the advertising propaganda and what we're told. A better distinction is between the heavy, grainy, dense loaf of centuries gone and the attractive but nutritional junk that passes for a bloomer, bap or baguette today.

Modern bread is a different thing entirely to what Chaucer knew in the Middle Ages. It's different even to the bread your grandmother ate as a child; with less gluten and more fibre it didn't instantly turn to sugar as soon as it reached her stomach – it also had *some* beneficial nutrients floating around in it.

After World War II, plant breeders developed new strains of wheat that delivered higher yields with the intensive applications of nasty substances, such as artificial nitrogen, herbicides and pesticides.

Because they wanted bigger yields and bigger profits, bakers included more stretchy protein molecules (gluten) while reducing the density of vital minerals and vitamins in the grain.

> *"The health of nations is more important*
> *than the wealth of nations."*
> **Will Durant**

Consequently, modern wheat strains are 30 to 40 per cent poorer in minerals such as iron, zinc and magnesium than the wheat eaten in the first half of the last century.

In the 1960s, bread took another turn for the worse when a new process (the 'Chorleywood Process') meant that loaves could be produced without having to wait the best part of a day for the yeast to rise.

Traditional methods of baking used to allow time for the dough to ripen and to neutralise some of the wheat protein most likely to trigger bowel disease and other auto-immune and inflammatory conditions. In the rush toward productivity, modern bread producing methods don't do this at all, and so this bread presents an even more serious challenge for the body to metabolise properly.

Because these new breads were being made so quickly, there was no longer sufficient time given to ripening the dough, a process which makes it easier to handle and ensures it tastes good. In order to solve this problem, modern bread manufacturers use literally hundreds of additives to achieve these effects artificially.

These bread additives are derived from substances that no human would normally eat, but we were told they were safe until, one-by-one, scientists told us they weren't.

Almost at the point of despair, the industry found a new category of 'improvers' - additives based on industrial enzymes. These 'natural' sources of biological catalysts are sourced from cereals, mould, bacteria and even animal guts. They now routinely go into bread.

Today, enzymes are the dirty little secret the baking industry is very reluctant to talk about.

This is what a modern 'wholemeal' loaf contains:

*Wholemeal Flour, Water, Caramelised Sugar, Yeast, Fermented Wheat Flour, Salt, Vegetable Fat, Wheat Protein, **Emulsifiers:** E472e, E471, Soya Flour, **Flour Treatment Agent:** Ascorbic Acid (source: the back of any bag of bread)*

In fact this isn't the whole 'roll' call. The list of additives was so long and scary that the bread industry was given special dispensation to simply use the terms **'flour treatment agents'** and **'emulsifiers'** to cover their tracks, avoid putting customers off and perhaps ruining a whole 'slice' of the economy.

When it comes to grain, wheat-based bread is just the most graphic example of a bad bunch, and it's low-nutrient, high-carb, high-sugar and highly-additive filled products like this that you need to avoid in whatever forms they might appear.

All high-carbohydrate foods will mess you up to a greater or lesser extent

Although not all high-carb foods are unhealthy, I would still suggest that you avoid them, especially if you hope to lose weight. Here's why:

1. *You probably can't handle even healthy, starchy carbohydrates such as sweet potato or rice (wild is best) until you have repaired the damage the rest of the unhealthy carbs have done.*

2. *High-carb foods produce a sugar (glucose) rush to the bloodstream that the body fails to stabilise well. A failure to stabilise blood-sugar levels leads to an increased release of a hormone called insulin.*

3. *Insulin, a natural hormone, takes sugar out of your bloodstream and puts it into the muscles, but in the presence of too much high-carb fare (and too much sugar) it can't do its job properly. More and more insulin*

is required to complete the job as your body starts to resist its action. This is the start of **insulin resistance***, a state most of us are in and which exists as a half-way house between good health and full-blown* **type II diabetes.**

4. *Increased levels of insulin tell the body to* **store fat.**

In short, regular ingestion of most high-carb foods will sooner or later make you obese, unable to handle sugar well, and *incapable of metabolising fat properly as an energy source.* It may also, given a little more time, give you diabetes. Sometimes, it gives you diabetes *before* it makes you fat – if you're really unlucky!

The irony is that overweight people with faulty carbohydrate metabolisms are told (by doctors, by government officials, by dieticians) to eat more carbohydrates and less fat.

They duly do this. They reduce their fat intake and eat more carbs. (In the UK we have been doing this *en masse* for decades.)

The insulin trap

As a modern day hunter-gatherer, your body is hardwired to store fat in times of plenty for periods when there may be an absence of good calories around. This evolutionary adaptation meant that when our ancestors did not have access to the meats and other foods their bodies required, their main energy system (which ran mainly on fat) was still able to provide them with sustained energy. Any fat around the body could easily be broken down and used to supply their calorific needs.

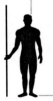

> What tasted best *was* best for our ancient ancestors. Our craving for Fat, Sweet and Salty flavours today is no unfortunate coincidence – it's these very deepest cravings that (like sex) kept our species going for millennia in an ancient world.

Stone Age man's palette was highly sensitised to the merest hint of sweetness or saltiness as this was his best indicator that a food would be high in fat and protein or nutrients. His taste buds would encourage him to consume meat whenever possible, or even certain sweet fruits, vegetables or honey (Before we started cultivating them, most vegetables were, although more nutritious, saddled with a sour taste.)

His love for sweet, salty or fatty foods discouraged him from choosing blander, less nutritional options like ground roots unless he had no other option. Given a choice between, say, bison and yams your body *wants* you to eat bison. It's no accident that in taste comparison tests, bison wins every time.

This drive for salty, sweet or fatty foods ensured our appetite remained fired up and able to motivate our behaviour towards hunting out our next nutritious meal.

Our sweet tooth once made us crave seasonal fruit or extremely limited supplies of honey. They were prized because of because of their nutritional value and, of course, their scarcity. These foods are now supplied year round by Tesco and other loveable supermarket chains, but the year-round purchase of fruit and honey from middle-ranking supermarkets isn't really the problem.

The real issue today is that modern foods are imposters. These pseudo-foods are capable of mimicking the tastes that we associate with healthy foods, while actually supplying us with something entirely different. They are a chimera, a poison chalice, a Trojan horse – use whatever metaphor you will.

Take breakfast cereal for example – any major brand. Even the ones that aren't frosted (covered in cheap sugar) affect our bodies in the way that no component of a Palaeolithic diet ever could.

As soon as the product reaches our mouths where – like sugar – it starts to digest very quickly, our taste buds are delighted they've been given something rare and sweet to feast on. Our instincts tell us that sweet things are special and should be eaten quickly while they're available. (Fruit and honey are a here today, gone tomorrow kind of thing in the wild. Not something you can depend on year round)

Cereal however, which to the brain tastes just the same (i.e. sweet and delicious), is much higher in carbohydrate content and available any time you want, year round. It starts to break down in the mouth very quickly, causing a rise the hormone, **insulin**, which takes glucose out of the bloodstream and into the muscles where it can be used as energy. However, the body can't handle this much sugar (as nothing exists like it in nature) so it requests more insulin than we were ever intended to produce to do the dirty job.

In a diet filled with this sort of high-calorie carbohydrate, the body is flooded with insulin on a long-term basis. Over time the muscles start to become de-sensitised and ignore the presence of insulin, and so stop taking this glucose into the muscles. This energy has got to go somewhere, so instead it is diverted and stored as fat.

The continual presence of all this sugar in the bloodstream raises blood sugar levels unnaturally high. The body is actually threatened by this and reacts by releasing adrenaline, giving the owner a temporary high.

However, what goes up must come down. When the individual finally takes a break from this cereal fest, his blood sugar levels crash, leading to instant fatigue, lethargy, premature sleepiness and sometimes depression (as with me in the bad old days). *This is prime fat storing time.*

Nobody likes feeling like this. Just like a junkie deprived of a hit, the body starts to crave another shot of adrenaline. Your appetite for foods with this taste is now thoroughly whetted. *"I'm so tired"* you tell yourself. *"Another bowl of cereal will give me the energy I need. After all, I felt on top of the world after the last one."* Our false reasoning only deepens the nutritional trap in which we have been so cleverly ensnared.

Boosted by our unrestrained instinct for more sweetness, salt or more fat, we start the cycle again; reaching for more food that our bodies continue to mistake for the occasional treat that nature offers (her fruit and honey) or the meat, fish or fowl which provides the calories in the form our body really needs: **fat!**

Taken to its furthest medical extreme this insidious process is responsible for **diabetes:** a state where the body is no longer able to produce insulin to control blood sugar levels at all. If not injected with a *man-made* insulin substitute, the glucose eventually builds up and crystallises in the blood doing irreparable damage to the circulatory system.

> The elephant in the room that no one seems to want to talk about is the fact that the real cause of both Type I and Type II diabetes and obesity is the abuse of modern processed carbohydrates.

Anyway, the result of this bad advice is that fat people take the advice they've been given and get inexorably fatter.

Friendly Fat

Fat, however, is the perfect fuel for us. If it wasn't, why would we store it around our bodies rather than starch or sugar? It is there because evolution decided it was the very *best* fuel to burn during lean times.

What people who have a phobia of body fat forget is that it is part of the grand design of our bodies. It evolved for a reason. Body fat doesn't just mean we've done something dumb or greedy. It's our body's defence against starving. Our bodies evolved the ability to put fat into cells for a reason - to store energy, which is fine. The issue is that many of us have too much of it, and have lost the ability to burn it off when we wish or need to.

The problem is that so many of us are simply too messed up to use our prime energy system. We don't consume much of it and we don't burn much of it. We're like a hybrid car that's stuck in one mode. Sedentary living, modern food toxins, too much stress and not enough sleep all contribute to this problem. (It's sometimes called 'Metabolic Syndrome' or 'Syndrome X').

> Most adults can't switch to burning stored fat; instead they run permanently on sugar (from sugar and carbs) in a way in which they were never 'designed' to.

By choosing animal fat as your primary fuel, you are returning to your ancestral human fuel source. And the best way to switch to fat burning is to start eating more meat (and low-carb veg) and whatever fat comes with that.

You'll come across people who will try to throw you off-track by telling you that they eat cheesecake every meal or McDonalds twice a day and still weigh the same as they did in college. And maybe they do. Maybe they've been lucky enough to get away without significant damage so far. Maybe they manage to run excess weight off with hours of cardio every week. Or maybe they actually haven't been so lucky; it's just not that plain to see yet. Not all poor health is visible around the waist. Wait twenty years and check back with them. The older someone gets, the more seriously you can take the evidence of their health claims.

On a personal note, I realised that I was getting skinny-fat when I was in my early thirties. Finally I made the high-carb connection and stopped eating what I now call 'peasant food' – pizza, pasta, bread, cakes, rice, potatoes and biscuits. In particular, I started avoiding gluten and I stuck to meat, fish, vegetables, fruit and nuts. Very quickly two things happened. I lost all the fat around my waist that had been building up over the previous four or five years and, amazingly, I discovered I was no longer tired or depressed after meals. Previously I had found that after most meals I felt like lying down to sleep for a few hours. I assumed I was eating too much. Because sleeping was often inconvenient, I was addicted to coffee to keep me going through the day.

After changing my diet I found that I could even eat large lunches and head into the afternoon full of energy. In fact, I had consistently high levels of energy through the day. These days I know myself well enough to know that if I opt for even a single sandwich, my body will protest and I will feel like heading to the sofa.

Interestingly, even when I knew that bread, pizza and the like was messing me up, I still craved it. It took me a while to realise that I was actually addicted to the sugar rush it produced and the adrenaline rush which accompanied my body's attempt to handle what it actually recognised as a threat. I just wish that I had recognised what was going on every day a little sooner.

Many of my clients tell me they couldn't go back to eating grains – wheat in particular – even if they wanted to. They say that it makes them feel so grotty now that it just isn't worth it. It seems that when we are consuming something regularly, even if it's bad for us, our bodies try to reduce our awareness of the symptoms; however, when we resume a harmful habit after a break from it, our body complains like never before in the hope of averting a return to previous bad habits. It seems that our bodies aren't as passive in this as we may have thought – and as we get healthier, we get more sensitive to unhealthy foods, not more able to tolerate them.

Non-Foods

It's not just the high-carb foods that need to be looked out for however. The western diet is now filled with substances which shouldn't really be dignified with the description 'food'. Many of these I can't mention by name as they come in so many guises and under many brand names (and I don't like being sued). However they have certain things in common; they often:

- *Come packaged in fancy boxes*
- *Have more than 3 or 4 ingredients (always a bad sign)*
- *Are pre-cooked*
- *Advertise some spuriously dubious feature (e.g. 'low fat', 'added iron')*
- *Are not actually a food (e.g. apple is a food; a Find-us crispy pancake is not – unless there's a pancake tree in nature that I'm unaware of…)*
- *Have long, silly names (e.g. 'I-can't-believe-we-sell-this-stuff-instead-of-butter')*

Vegetable Oil

This is an oil (though it is sometimes referred to as vegetable fat) made from the contents of highly-processed seeds. It's made from plants such as sunflower, corn, safflower, cottonseed, peanut or soybean and becomes a polyunsaturated fatty acid (PUFA). It is always heavily **Hydrogenated**, which simply means that it has been heated up to a temperature high enough that its actual molecular structure is damaged.

These **trans-fats** (as they are called) incite havoc in cell metabolism. Research indicates that trans-fats cause comparatively more weight gain than the same diet with monounsaturated oils and a lead to a redistribution of body fat tissue to the abdominal area, the riskiest place to carry extra padding. Additionally, they're associated with inflammation and atherosclerosis, the processes responsible for cancers, heart conditions and most other modern diseases.

They are so bad that even the establishment has had to acknowledge their pernicious effects. In New York and all of California they have been banned outright. Denmark was the first country to ban them and it is hypothesised that the Danish government's efforts to decrease trans-fat intake from 6g to 1g per day over 20 years is related to a 50% decrease in deaths from ischemic heart disease.

The UK food authorities are still fine with their use, however. You can still find hydrogenated vegetable oils in half the products in your local supermarket. Typically they'll be found in margarine, bread, pastries, donuts, muffins, biscuits, cookies, cakes, pies, crackers, chips, instant flavoured coffee drinks, microwave popcorn, and the usual fast food suspects like fried chicken and French fries.

As cooking oils, trans-fats are the number one choice of consumers – most of whom, presumably, are happily unaware that they are using a product that is so rancid that it has to have perfumes added to it so that the smell does not deter consumption.

In the UK, most people still think that margarine, which is made from highly-concentrated vegetable oil trans-fat, is a preferable alternative to butter. Oops!

Once you start reading labels, you'll realise this stuff is everywhere. So much mixed-ingredient food is contaminated with the stuff.

So why do manufacturers use it? Well it's about profit again, of course. Trans-fats[2] produce a crispy, flaky feel to food and extend it beyond its natural shelf-life. Customers, unless they are biologists or nutritionists, have little idea what they are actually eating. Producers are forced by law to print this information on their labels, but I'm sure it hasn't missed your notice that they do a fine job of disguising the truth in the tiniest writing, ambiguous E numbers, and various other forms of devious sneakery.

If you're looking for a really evil enemy to vent your fury against in the context of modern illness, look primarily at this spiteful, nasty toxic matter. I would list this as public health enemy number one, even above modern grains (which are usually mixed with these trans-fats/hydrogenated vegetable oils in a processed form anyway).

A 2004 study by Brigham and Women's Hospital and Harvard School of Public Health showed that in postmenopausal women, the more PUFA they ate and, to a much lesser extent, the more carbohydrate they ate, the worse their atherosclerosis (hardening of the arteries) became over time. Interestingly, the more saturated fat they ate, the less their atherosclerosis progressed; in the group with the highest intake of saturated fat, the atherosclerosis actually reversed over time.[3]

Omegas 3 & 6

You've probably heard by now about Omegas 3 and 6. In health circles, Omega 6 is currently the villain of the story and Omega 3 very much the darling heroine. Omegas are types of fatty acids found in polyunsaturated fat. PUFAs are mostly found in nuts, seeds, fish, algae, and leafy greens. In their denatured form they are found in almost all processed food.

You may have seen your doctor or watched something on the news and wondered whether you're getting enough Omega 3 in your diet. If you're not, it may be suggested that you increase your intake of Omega 3s by eating seafood twice a week or by taking a fish oil supplement.

This is sound advice.

The presence of **hydrogenated vegetable oil** (a seed-based PUFA) in so many foods has meant that our diet has become heavily unbalanced in favour of Omega 6. In the hydrogenation process (when the oil is super-heated) the actual molecular structure of the oil is damaged. It then suffers further damage through oxidation in storage before we consume it.

It is thought that optimal health demands a ratio of 1:1 or 2:1 or maybe a high as 4:1 in favour of Omega 6[4], but modern western diets typically have ratios of in excess of 10 to 1, some as high as 30 to 1. Omega 6 competes with Omega 3. Because it's the ratio that's important[3], eating more Omega 3 will cancel out a certain proportion of Omega 6s consumed. However, most of us are consuming damaged Omega 6s with such abandon that even eating fish AND adding a fish oil (like cod liver) is unable to rebalance the ratio.

Excess Omega 6 is associated with all modern inflammatory conditions[5], particularly:

- Asthma
- Arthritis
- Vascular disease
- Thrombosis
- Immune-inflammatory processes
- Tumour proliferation
- Heart attacks
- Arrhythmia, arthritis
- Osteoporosis
- Inflammation
- Mood disorders
- Obesity and cancer

You can see, therefore, how counterproductive frying your weekly meal of fish in vegetable oil to cancel out the effects of the previous night's processed meal would be!

There are other ingredients to look out for besides vegetable oil as soon as you stray into the product aisles; this comes down to reading the labels.

Look out for foods with:

- **Added sugar** – *Any additional sugar in your diet adds to the same problem as high-carbs – a swamping of the glucose energy system with instantly available energy, which leads to excess insulin, which leads to* *body fat retention. It also deranges your palate so that you can no longer enjoy the subtler taste of good food.*

● **Added salt** – *this is always in the form of table salt (sodium). Table salt has been stripped of all of the useful minerals that are found in natural rock salt or sea salt. An excess of this can affect your blood pressure.*

● **Added starches** – *e.g. corn starch, tapioca starch. These produce the same problems as grain consumption.*

● **Artificial colouring and flavouring** – *known as E numbers. You'll have read about the dangers of these before. They are implicated in conditions such as ADHD, and mood and behavioural disorders, especially in childhood.*

● **Artificial sweeteners** – *These have many names, such as: fructose, sucrose, dextrose, maltodextrin, aspartame – even eating tablespoons of sugar is better than consuming these harmful alternatives. Fizzy drinks, sports drinks and most protein powders are rife with this stuff. All sugar substitutes other than stevia are made from this stuff. The long term effect of consumption is still a huge, dangerous unknown, but they are potentially carcinogenic according to some health researchers.*

● **Excess caffeine** – *A cup or two of organic coffee a day is ok, but heavily-caffeinated 'energy' drinks will disrupt your entire metabolism and hormonal balance. Excess caffeine can also be used to mask energy imbalances and disrupted blood sugar levels. Avoid.*

● **Soya** – *Is grain-like and contains lectins, Phytates and Phytoestrogens. The latter increase the production of the oestrogen hormone, producing 'moobs' in men. The quantities of this found in vegetarians' diets is just one more reason to avoid being one if you can.*

"SAT FAT"

If seed oil is SO bad, then what alternatives are there, you will want to know. The answer is lots!

Organic butter, ghee, lard, coconut oil, tallow, left-over bacon fat – any of these. (Olive oil is fine too, as long as you avoid damaging it with excess heat.) However, as I discussed earlier in the book, you've probably been warned off these for the last 50 years because they contain *saturated fat*.

The pop science explanation of the 'dangers' of saturated fat goes something like this:

> *"Y'see, when you eat fatty foods, especially those rich in animal fat, the saturated fat and cholesterol in these foods wind up in your blood and stick to your arteries. 'Cos saturated fats are solid outside your body, they will be solid inside your body too* (er, despite the 30-degree increase in average temperature?). *Arteries are much like pipes. When they get caked up with grease, blood flow is impaired, and a heart attack ensues."*

This simple, primary-school-level explanation has caught hold of the public's imagination because it's so easy to understand with its 'think-about-why-your-sink-gets-blocked' analogy. It is, however, absolute nonsense. Not even the early scientists who set this anti-sat-fat train rolling had a notion of science that was this fundamentally wrong. Their explanation, although also incorrect, was at least partially logical and valid, unlike the popular notions that have stopped most people enjoying a substance that our bodies evolved to use as their major fuel.

Even mothers' breast milk is 50% fat, much of it saturated. Any biologist can tell you that saturated fat and cholesterol are essential to a baby's growth.

However, we are told to believe that it somehow becomes deadly as we get older. Does that make sense to you?

Standby – here comes some science…

As I hope I've made clear by now, almost all modern disease is caused by excessive inflammation and oxidisation. Cholesterol is made of two types: LDL (bad cholesterol) and HDL (good cholesterol). Cardio-vascular disease, more specifically, seems to be caused by oxidised LDL. (You can think of oxidisation as internal 'rusting'.) Research is showing fairly conclusively that the rise in the prevalence of LDL is associated with modern inflammatory conditions.

Oxidised LDL initiates the inflammatory process by causing cells to secrete molecules that attract T cells and other inflammatory

---

cells. The question arises of what causes LDL to oxidise in the first place. Since PUFAs in the LDL membrane are the components that are most vulnerable to oxidation, excess PUFAs and insufficient antioxidants (the sort found in vegetables and fruit) would seem to be the most obvious culprits.

Oxidisation causes the production of free radicals[6] which make their way through the body attacking everything in sight. The damage takes a toll on everything from cell membranes to DNA to blood vessels, which then lead to plaque accumulation. The harm adds up over time in the organs and systems of the body, and can cause a significant impact, including premature aging, skin disease, liver damage, immune dysfunction, and even cancer.

Don't worry if you didn't follow all of the above. In real terms, *we are eating too much industrial seed oil* (like sunflower, corn, canola, soybean oils) while failing to eat enough vegetables to offset the damage.

By now you'll be getting a pretty good idea of what, from an evolutionary point of view, is good to eat. There are lots – I mean hundreds – of alternative 'diets' out there that if you fall for the hype will take you seriously off track. Most fad diets today have been built upon the received wisdom of accepted nutritional science (low fat, high carb), so they try in vain to twist the accepted facts into 'new' more palatable and marketable models. As soon as you move away from the principle that we should eat what we evolved to eat, any nutrition advice becomes increasingly hard to justify.

Here is a very brief overview of the main 'wonder' diets that have appeared recently:

Low-fat diets

I think we've dealt with this already. Low-fat means that to get the calories your body needs, you must turn to extra grain and heavy-carbs as an alternative source of calories. It also often means processed instant meals with nasty ingredients.

Low-calorie diets

Leaping into bed with the government's low-fat advice is the **super-low-calorie** approach to weight-loss. If you remember though, our bodies have been programmed by evolution to try to hang onto fat when threatened by the possibility of running short of nutrients or fat to burn. When you cut the calories, your body feels threatened and will try to retain the fat it already has. Instead, the weight you lose (if any) will be in the form of excess water (we're made of 60% water of course) and depleted muscle mass.

Weightwatchers (WW) is the classic example of this. This multi-national company founded its credentials on the idea that eating fewer kilo-calories of energy by sticking to WW's 'low-fat' meals is a great way to lose weight. It's low-calorie by dint of the fact that the meals are low in sugar (good), low in salt (good) and low in fat (bad). (They're also low in nutrients by the way too).

Sticking with the WW's plan (and it's not easy) means you will certainly lose weight but you will *lose muscle as well as any fat.* Muscle actually consumes calories during the day, so having lost muscle, the same number of calories you used to consume will make you fatter than you used to be as fewer calories will be consumed by your muscle mass. Since no one can eat like this for very long (long-term hunger hurts!) you will inevitably go back to your old habits and put all the weight back on again – *and more besides.* If you're smart you will conclude that WW doesn't work; if you're dumb you will reason that things were fine when you were with WW, so you'll sign up for a few more months of misery.

This low-calorie/low-fat approach is really widespread now, despite the fact that it clearly doesn't work. "Just eat less and exercise more" we are told by condescending, ignorant, overweight, hypocritical government ministers. If it were that simple, everybody could do it and nobody would need to write books about it.

There are no books, for example, about changing light bulbs, as far as I know. That's because it's relatively easy. There are loads of books about diets, because almost none of them work for people in the long term. 90%

of them are variations of the idea of eating less food/fat/calories – and fail to take account of the way that the body handles different sorts of foods or our instinctive biological drives.

Vegetarianism/veganism

Gosh, this one's a real can of worms. Suffice to say that humans evolved to eat meat. There really isn't any serious debate about this, although you wouldn't believe it if you stray onto a vegetarian website. Here you will read that we are actually so much like primates that we should still be eating fruit, as that's what apes eat. Oh, and we should eat vegetables and grains because apes also eat… oh no, they don't do they? Well I'm not sure entirely how their argument hangs together. They also like to conveniently miss out the fact that chimpanzees, our nearest living evolutionary cousins, also eat meat in the form of smaller primates.

To be fair, vegetarianism can produce some good results, such as if somebody opts for it instead of eating the usual rounds of McDonald's, vegetable-oil-cooked-MSG-filled Chinese meals, pork pies and crisps. Pretty much everybody will feel better under those circumstances. The problem is that the vegetarian diet is not a safe long-term option. It is simply too low in protein and healthy fat, and alternatives to meat are just not adequate.

Vegetarians often end up eating huge quantities of tofu and soya, neither of which are healthy replacements.[7] They also have to consume a lot of grain to keep hunger at bay. Vegetarians are usually weak and spindly or kind of fat; rarely do you see one with low-levels of fat and a reasonable, healthy amount of muscle.

Paleo v Vegetarian Ethics

Some vegetarians will tell you that they have chosen their diet because the consumption of meat and dairy is unsustainable and can't be a staple for 7 billion people. This seems to me an arguable point, but I would say that it is a high-carbohydrate, high-grain diet that has allowed the world's population to grow to a point where it seems we cannot sustain everyone with healthy foods. Is the answer for everyone to continue to eat unhealthily so that the world's population can continue to grow ad infinitum? I don't think so.

However, this is all beside the point. I am not an economist, but I don't think I'm wrong when I say that the reason that parts of the world do not have enough to eat is because of *poverty* – a failure to distribute resources adequately – not a lack of grain production.

As far as animal welfare goes, responsible Paleo eating involves choosing local produce that comes from well-treated animals which have lived healthy, happy lives. Large-scale industrial farming is another thing entirely and should not be put in the same bracket.

Low GI diets

This is actually quite sensible. The GI (Glycaemic Index) is a measure of how quickly a food breaks down into glucose and enters the bloodstream. Bread, for example is given a rating of about 75, whereas sweet potato is given a rating of about 54. Both of these foods are carbohydrates, starchy and high in calories, but the sweet potato is the better choice because it will not produce the same elevated blood sugar levels (and corresponding insulin levels) that (nasty, modern) bread will.

My only criticism of the diet is that while it's okay for weight loss, it's not necessarily healthy. There are foods filled with grain and processed nastiness which, according to the numbers, should result in weight-loss but actually won't as they cause an increased inflammatory response which is counter-productive for both weight loss and improved good health. For example, malt loaf is quite low in the GI index but can't be recommended for weight loss or better health.

The Atkins Diet

Poor old, much-maligned Atkins. Say what you will about him, but it cannot be denied that people who followed his diet (a diet, if you believe what people say, consisting of nothing but meat and eggs) lost A LOT of weight. Protein and fat is *very* satiating, so it's hardly surprising that people ended up eating fewer calories without really meaning to. Adherents also didn't lose too much muscle mass either (unlike turning vegetarian or going super-low calorie) as the higher protein diet provided all the building blocks they needed to maintain muscle mass.

His meat/egg/fish heavy diet was criticised by the establishment for eschewing 'healthy' carbs (like bread!) and encouraging the consumption of 'dangerously high' levels of saturated fat. When he contracted cardiomyopathy in 2000, a vegan group (with a drum to beat) put about a lot of false rumours that his heart condition was diet related. Some of the mainstream media were quick to use this as evidence of the unhealthiness of his diet.

In fact, his doctor said at the time that there was no evidence that his diet contributed to the condition. His cardiologist stated that (other than the cardiomyopathy), Atkins had "an extraordinarily healthy cardiovascular system". His coronary arteries were checked at that time and found to be free of blockages.

Much of what Atkins proposed was eminently sensible. He is sometimes criticised for not placing enough emphasis on the consumption of fresh vegetables, but even this may be a misrepresentation of the full Atkins plan which reinstated vegetables after only a few weeks of withdrawal. Unfortunately, in phases 4 and 5, it also reinstated grains, had no concern about meat quality and allowed the consumption of Omega 6 damaged vegetable oils and artificial sweeteners. Oh well, no one's perfect…

(Interestingly it seems that human beings *can* actually live on meat alone. Indeed, certain tribes, both ancient and modern, have done so for thousands of years. The Inuit for example as discussed earlier, live of a diet of almost nothing but saturated blubber from seals, whales, etcetera, year round. However, there is a caveat: to get all the nutrients, vitamins and minerals and anti-oxidants that a diet rich in vegetables would provide, you have to eat the *whole* animal – brains, liver, kidneys, bone marrow - everything. Not many of us are prepared to do this of course, so vegetables remain a tasty, nutritious and pretty much unavoidable component of a good diet.)

Fasting

"Fat people who want to reduce should take their exercise on an
empty stomach and sit down to their food out of breath...
Thin people who want to get fat should do exactly the opposite
and never take exercise on an empty stomach."

Hippocrates

Some diets focus on simply not eating. For thousands of years fasting has been an important part of people's lives. For the hunter-gatherer, fasting was an inescapable fact of life when access to food proved irregular. For many civilisations that followed, deliberate fasting was an established religious, social and health practice. There are multitudinous reasons for this, but in almost every culture bar our own fasting has been used as a gateway to superior emotional, spiritual or physical health. There may be no other culture that is as scared to deprive itself of food, even temporarily, than ours.

Moreover, science has recently revealed that when the body is deprived of food entirely it produces very specific changes in its chemistry.

Brief fasting reduces oxidative stress (it's a de-tox), improves insulin sensitivity (which is great for weight loss) and improves protein uptake (for building muscle). Even better, a period of hunger actually turns on the body's anti-ageing mechanism.

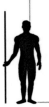

In thousands of trials with mice, only calorie restriction has consistently shown to extend average and maximum life spans: and it does so by between 30 to 50 per cent! What we've only just discovered is that these same benefits can be enjoyed by humans, even if they fast only for short periods of time.

I've already spent some time criticising low-calorie diets so you might think that fasting is merely an extreme version of the same. However the science suggests that *short* periods of fasting can produce all the benefits looked at above without the slower metabolism or muscle loss that long-term low-calorie diets (and long-term fasting) produce.

Perhaps one of the biggest threats we have to contend with these days is the lack of variability in calories consumed from day to day. We evolved to eat as much as we can, just as often as we can – which was much of the time, but not *all* the time. Sometimes we would just have to go without, and doing so benefits the body in ways that a continual, monotonous supply of calories doesn't.

On occasion our ancestors would have hunted (exercised /walk/sprinted) vigorously without success. They would have often exercised on an empty stomach - sometimes more than once before having the chance to consume significant calories.

This meant that they became adapted to providing energy from stored body fat while maintaining steady blood glucose levels. Any fasted exercise they did forced them to dip into their fat reserves – hence there was always a serious absence of fat cavemen. By way of contrast, we have almost all been taught to 'fuel-up' before exercise. The result of this is that we must burn through glucose and glycogen supplies in the body before we can begin using any fat as fuel. This is the simple reason that most people don't lose much weight even when they start an exercise programme. In fact, because they are unused to having low glucose levels in their blood, they will almost always eat more carbohydrate after exercise to make up for the increased hunger they experience. Hence regular exercisers can often get fatter!

I hope you now understand why in **Chapter 10** I'll recommend that you miss a meal or two a week to disrupt the usual 3-or-more-meals-a-day (plus snacks) routine that most of us fall into.

By undertaking the occasional fast you will:

- *massively kick-start weight-loss*
- *encourage anti-aging mechanisms*
- *improve immune system defences*
- *stabilise blood-sugar levels*
- *improve hormonal balances.*

From an evolutionary standpoint, it's imperative that your body gets the signal that calories are *sometimes* in short supply so you can continue to thrive as an organism.

Your genes are pretty selfish: They care little about you, and only care about their own survival; initially through you, then later and more crucially through your offspring. When calories are abundant, your body concerns itself less with extending your longevity, as it will assume that your progeny will survive to pass on your genes.

Nasty genes!

You'll notice that this chapter is longer than all the others. That's because I consider it perhaps the most important. The other two elements of Instinctive Fitness: **Natural Movement** and **Natural Lifestyle** are also massively important, but if this pillar is not addressed, the other stuff just doesn't matter so much.

You'll realise by now that I am not so much proposing a diet as an eating style, focusing on *what* to eat, rather than how much.

In terms of body composition (or just 'looking great naked', if you prefer) eating the right foods is 80% of the battle. It really doesn't matter if you are an aspiring bodybuilder (!), want to look like Bruce Lee or Megan Fox, *or* just want to lose that paunch – it really is all about the food.

That said, you want to avoid becoming totally hung up on eating - counting calories, measuring your food, or other neurotic things like weighing yourself daily. No self-respecting cavemen ever weighed themselves!

The plan should be dead simple. Here it is:

- *Start by eliminating all the offensive, processed food, grains, sugar and industrial oils.*
- *Eat meat, seafood, eggs, vegetables, fruit, nuts, herbs and spices, healthy oils.*
- *Eat two or three times a day – no more.*

I should say a little about each of these though to guide you in your selection and nudge you towards quality. *Every bit of extra income you spend on improving the quality of your food is the best investment in your future you can make.*

Meat

Go for organic and/or local meats whose flesh comes from animals free from injected growth hormones, antibiotics and other stimulants. Choose anything from beef, pork, lamb, chicken, venison, quail, duck, turkey, and other whole meat products. Wild game is great. Salami, spam and processed ham are out! Liver, kidneys and other organ meat is superlative and contain certain vitamins that are hard to get elsewhere. Organic bacon is wonderful and, now you've got over your 'sat-fat' fears, can be demolished without guilt at your leisure.

Omega 6s: try to buy beef (or whatever) that is **100% grass-fed** ('pasture fed'). I can't emphasise this enough. Cows should eat grass (I expect you know this, and perhaps didn't realise most cows today don't) *not* grain. For cows in many modern industrial farms where they consume a concentrated diet of corn, grain and soy, their flesh is dominated by excessive Omega 6 PUFAs, large quantities of antibiotics (needed to counteract their unnatural diet), and a high level of growth hormones.

> While this sorry state of affairs continues in industrial farming, perhaps the government is right to recommend that most people restrict the amount of meat they eat!

Buy meat produced locally. Even if you're not interested in the ecological arguments (transportation costs, fuel consumption, air pollution, etc.) or the ethical arguments (about inhumane travelling conditions for animals), the fact is that local food arrives in a much fitter state for consumption than that which comes from the other side of the country or abroad. Animals that have been well-treated have much lower levels of stress hormones, and that improves the quality of their meat considerably.

Supermarkets sell food that is a lot older than you might expect and by the time you consume it it has only a fraction of the nutrients you need.

Look into local suppliers, ideally straight from a local farm. www.bigbarn. co.uk will give you some idea where to start if you want to take this road.

I think that it is kinder to give your custom to farms that keep their animals outside for most of the year rather those that house them on top of each other in enormous barns where they have no contact with nature and little room to move.

Fish and Seafood

Choose **wild fish**, *never* fish that has been farmed. Farmed fish is higher in Omega 6 and contains less protein. Farmed fish also comes with dioxins, (cancer-linked) PCBs, fire retardants (!), pesticides (especially for sea lice), antibiotics, copper sulphate (to take care of algae on the nets), and canthaxanthin (a dye to make grey farmed fish various shades of "wild" pink). If you do eat farmed fish, environmental groups suggest you eat no more than one serving per month. That tells you all you need to know about farmed fish!

Eggs

Choose **local free-range** eggs, of course. Ideally 'pasture fed' and organic. Don't sponsor the madness that keeps hens shut up in tiny cages for their whole lives. Even if you don't care about this, the lower quality of egg (and their higher quantity of Omega 6) is more than enough reason to avoid eggs from caged-hens.

You should look for chickens that have a chance to get outside during the day and, ideally, forage for their own food. It is okay if they have been fed some grain as chickens (unlike cattle) have a digestive system that is properly equipped to process the stuff. However, chickens are at their best when they are digging around for bugs, worms and other bits of protein. If you can buy from someone who keeps their chickens like this and avoid supermarket fare, you're doing really well.

Free-range is almost a given these days amongst thinking people who aren't on the breadline (a well-chosen phrase as I'd have to be desperate before I bought supermarket bread!). What's ironic though is that many people who wouldn't consider buying anything other than free-range, actually eat plenty of battery-farmed eggs in all the processed food them consume!

Vegetables

Eat lots of them. They should fill up more than half the space on your plate. Choose lots of different coloured vegetables (as silly as that sounds) as the different colours denote different types of vitamins and anti-oxidants. "Eat the rainbow, man" - as they like to say in the US.

Due to their nutritional profile, green vegetables (spinach, broccoli, kale, lettuce, seaweed, etc.) are of particular importance.

Potatoes are, of course, also a vegetable, but they were bred to be starchy in the New World and so won't help in weight-loss and don't offer much in terms of good nutrition. When you reach your ideal 'fighting weight', and you have moved away from being a perennial, sugar-burning 'carb-head', you might like to opt for sweet potato (which is lower on the G.I. scale).

Vegetables are where you are going to pick up many of the vitamins you need to live healthily, to keep a strong immune system, and to delay the on-set of premature ageing. This is the secret hidden in plain view. Buying organic not only avoids contaminants from the farming process, but also produces a product that is richer in nutrients than those grown in our increasingly mineral-depleted soils.

If you're hoping for a 'miracle' recovery from serious disease, you could start by looking at nine portions of vegetables a day. Watch Dr Terry Wahls in "Minding Your Mitochondria" on YouTube for an eye-opening personal account of the power of vegetables.

Again ideally buy *local organic vegetables* which will be far fresher and freer from contaminants, pesticides and herbicides.

Fruits

Most fruits are great and confer the same amazing health-giving properties as vegetables – especially seasonal, local, high quality stuff. They are, however, heavier on sugar. These fruits are not quite the same products as those our forest-dwelling ancestors would have eaten, which would have been more sour and fibrous. This only starts to make much of difference if you start chugging fruit juices by the carton or eating one banana after another. (Bananas are quite carb heavy – beware!). If you must drink fruit juice, make sure it's not 'from concentrate' and dilute it with water as much as you can. Avoid dried fruits because they are filled with sugar; they're natural, but fattening.

Nuts

A bit like fruit: great in moderation. There's no doubt they are a healthy, natural food, filled with B vitamins and essential minerals like magnesium, calcium, potassium, zinc and iron. If you've eaten a small handful to reach a meal, such as a late evening meal, to avoid your still-stabilising blood sugar levels dropping too low, that's fine.

If you are necking them by the packetful every day, you are going to be consuming a lot of very dense calories which may seriously impede weight-loss. Some are also rather high in Omega 6s. Make sure they are not coated in sugar or vegetable oil. The best nut is the macadamia; these are so packed full of nutrients they can almost be considered a super food. By the way, despite their misleading name, peanuts are not a nut; they are a legume in disguise - avoid.

Salad oils and cooking oils

Use olive oil for salad dressing (it's not a seed-oil). Cook meat and vegetables with any sort of animal fat, or butter. Goose fat is great, as is coconut oil. Avoid heating olive oil up much as it degrades in the same way as mass-produced, rancid, dangerous vegetables oils that are damaged in the hydrogenation process. Store it at room temperature in the dark. *Remember that fat is needed for the body to absorb vitamins A, D, E and K, so we cut it out of our diets at our peril!*

Okay-in-moderation foods

In this category, I would include a few items that are health-giving in some ways but whose disadvantages could easily outweigh the benefits if they are overindulged in. Also, some these items are best avoided in the early days while weight-loss is still a priority. There are also a handful of items that aren't really Paleolithic in chronology but which, on balance, might not be too harmful if consumed sensibly. (This plan is about gaining benefits, not about recreating a historical period in time.)

Examples of these would be:

Chocolate - dark only, 70% cocoa or more. Avoid for weight-loss but it does contain high levels of anti-oxidants to combat free radicals. Buy fair-trade if you're nice.

Red wine - Of all alcohols, red wine confers the most advantages. Like chocolate, it contains very high levels of anti-oxidants and, in moderation, is good for reducing stress. Consider two small glasses a day your limit though!

Tea and coffee - High levels of caffeine contribute to stress, high cortisone levels and skyward blood sugar levels; however, a cup or two of coffee or tea a day will do no harm. Non-organic coffee contains some of the highest levels of pesticide and herbicide of any household products, so always buy **organic**. Though classed as a stimulant, tea or coffee is always preferable to fizzy drinks, chemical-filled beers or grain-based spirits.

Honey - It turns out that eating local, raw, cloudy honey made from your local pollens may reduce hay fever symptoms by boosting your body's immunity (at least for as long as you remain in your region).[8] It's quite sugar-laden, so, even though it's natural sugar, you won't win any slimmer of the month awards if you feast on this year round. But as local honey is seasonal, you can't – see how clever nature is?

Healthy, heavier carbs

Foods are included under this heading because if you jump at these products before you have lost the weight you want to, *you will not reach your ideal weight.* Examples of healthy higher carbs that you can consume once your metabolism has recovered are **wild rice** (which is a grass, not a grain), **sweet potato, parsnips, quinoa and buckwheat** (which is technically a seed-based food).

You also might include some of these in your *transition* to a lower-carb eating plan as they can help avoid any temporary 'fug' or energy lag as your body switches to burning fat (and internal glucose), rather than the high-carb stuff it's accustomed to. People who keep excess weight off easily or those more interested in muscle gain than weight-loss might include some of these items too. This sort of food is not essential for endurance events, however; no matter what Conventional Wisdom will tell you, "Carbo Loading" is never required.

Dairy - This is a difficult one and a hotly disputed topic. Again it probably comes down to product quality and people's individual differences. Some people simply don't do well on milk, cheese and other dairy products. Some people find that when they cut these things out of their diet, long-standing eczema conditions (or whatever else was troubling them) clear up within a week. Other people, however, seem to run on the stuff just fine.

Strictly speaking, Paleo is anti-dairy; however, I think the best policy is to cut dairy out of your diet for a month. Then, if all seems good, reintroduce it suddenly and heavily and note the effects. You might need to test cheese and milk separately. Like a good scientist, try not to change any other factors at the same time. If it seems to make no difference, then you're probably fine with dairy.

Having said that, there are a few stipulations if you are going to enjoy milk and cheese. First, always go for **full-fat**. *Semi-skimmed and skimmed milk is more heavily processed and is damaged in the heating process* (rather like vegetable oil). It also doesn't contain the energy that you need to replace the heavy-carb you've now forsaken. Always choose **organic** milk or, if you can get it (and this is the holy nectar of milk), drink **raw milk**. There is virtually no health risk with this if you get it from an established supplier. (Yes, it is legal. Search Google for your nearest farmer who makes deliveries). Alternatively, **Guernsey and Jersey milk** (Gold Top) is superior to ordinary milk if you don't mind the richer taste. Personally, I love it in coffee.

If you buy cheese, then look for **raw cheeses,** which are unpasteurised and therefore keep their goodness.

A warning!

Although I've just listed a number of tasty foods to be enjoyed in moderation, please don't forget that the bulk of your calories needs to come from animals, eggs, fish and meat, along with plenty of vegetables. Only if you make this your focus will you end up with the health benefits and the body composition characteristics you are aiming for. Remember to get the basics right first! You are going to make a radical change in altering your main fuel from carbs to fat – a change your body will continue to thank you for for the rest of your life, so don't compromise the benefits by looking for every easy indulgence you can find an excuse to consume before you've even got any steam up.

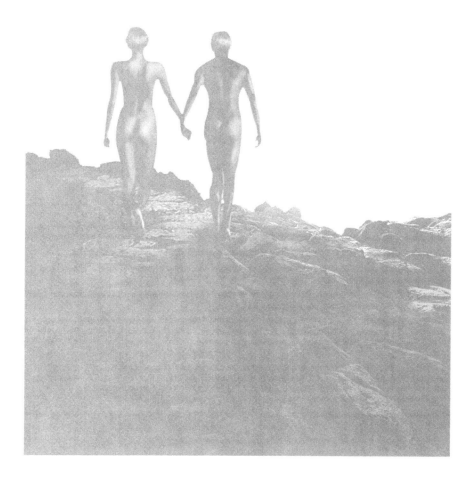

Key Chapter Points

- *"Eat Naturally Edible Food" – organic/grass-fed meat, wild fish, eggs, local/organic vegetables, fruit, nuts, herbs and spices, and healthy oils.*

- *Don't eat grains, sugar, starches, margarines, vegetable oils, or industrially-processed foods.*

- *Balance your Omegas, by eating more wild fish and avoiding noxious, processed foods (especially vegetable oils).*

- *Avoid all high-carb fare (even rice and sweet potato) until you've lost excess fat.*

- *Instead, get your energy from additional sources of fat, especially saturated fat (but avoid trans-fats!).*

- *Don't starve yourself to lose weight (it won't work in the long term). However, missing a meal and exercising instead once or twice a week will massively kick-start fat loss.*

- *Eat two or three times a day – no more.*

- *Buy the best quality, organic, free-range, local, grass-fed food you can afford.*

References:

1. Cuatrecasas P, Tell GPE (1973) "Insulin-Like Activity of Concanavalin A and Wheat Germ Agglutinin—Direct Interactions with Insulin Receptors." Department of Medicine, The Johns Hopkins University School of Medicine

2. Stender S, Dyerberg J (2004). "Influence of trans fatty acids on health". Ann. Nutr. Metab. 48(2):61–66.

3. Mozaffarian D, Rimm EB, Herrington DM. (2004) "Dietary fats, carbohydrate, and progression of coronary atherosclerosis in postmenopausal women." Am J Clin Nutr, 80(5): 1175-1184.

4. Eaton SB, Eaton SB 3rd, Sinclair AJ, Cordain L, Mann NJ (1998) "Dietary intake of long-chain polyunsaturated fatty acids during the Paleolithic Period." World Rev Nutr Diet, 12-23.

5. Kinsella JE (1988) Food Technology 134; Lasserre M et al (1985) "Effects of different dietary intake of essential fatty acids on C20:3 omega 6 and C20:4 omega 6 serum levels in human adults." Lipids 20(4):227; also Simopoulos AP (2002) "The importance of the ratio of omega-6/omega-3 essential fatty acids." Biomed Pharmacother, 56(8):365-379.

6. Machlin IJ, Bendich A, (1987) "Interesterification." FASEB Journal, 1:441-445 [Online] Available at: http://www.westonaprice.org/know-your-fats/556-interesterification.html; Enig, MG (1995) Trans Fatty Acids in the Food Supply: A Comprehensive Report Covering 60 Years of Research, 2nd Edition, Enig Associates, Inc, Silver Spring, MD, 148-154; Enig MG et al (1990) "Isomeric trans fatty acids in the U.S. diet." J Am Coll Nutr, 9(5):471-486.

7. The Weston A. Price Foundation (2012) "Soy Alert!" [Online] Available at: http://www.westonaprice.org/soy-alert.html.

8. Saarinen K, Jantunen J, Haahtela T. (2011) "Birch pollen honey for birch pollen allergy--a randomized controlled pilot study." Int Arch Allergy Immunol, 155(2):160-166.

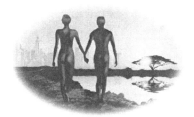

CHAPTER SEVEN

"Instinctive Fitness" - A Third Way

"The wise man sees in the misfortune of
others what he himself should avoid"

Marcus Aurelius
(Roman Emperor 121-180)

I think it's pretty much a given that everyone 'knows' they should be fit and healthy, and nearly everyone *wants* to be fit and healthy. Some people put the care and maintenance of their body at the centre of their lifestyle: open-mindedly exploring what works best for them. Others are more like I used to be: blindly going through the motions we've been told are right and not noticing we're getting nowhere fast.

For the vast majority of the population, health and fitness are seen as a chore to be avoided or a luxury continually pushed down the list of priorities. The following categories are generalisations and few people fit neatly into just one camp, but I think people can be neatly divided into two groups.

1. The sedentary time bomb (Doesn't – or tries not to - care)

The first option is filled with apathetic individuals who are generally doing nothing other than what life actively demands. This means that, for the most part, they are taking it easy, moving very little at all and indulging heavily in 'bait foods' that fool us with their attractive but manufactured appearance and taste.

These people take the common position of assuming that if everyone else does little exercise and eats foods full of sugar and starch, then it's okay for them to do so too (as long as the saturated fats are kept under control of course!)

This may be OK for the first few decades of life, but as the years and pounds roll on – heart disease, diabetes, cancer and all the other health monsters wait patiently in the wings before arriving on stage to pay their respects.

2. The Fitness Martyr ('No pain, no gain')

The second option is for people who not only *want* to be in better shape – but are actually prepared to do something about it. This is a path the vast majority seem to take. On and off at least. Usually set off by listening to a friend, reading a magazine or buying a book or DVD that spurs them into action, this person has all the best intentions to shape up!

So they roll up their sleeves and prepare themselves for the hard slog they're going to put themselves through. This new found enthusiasm usually lasts a few weeks or even months, usually with one sole intention in mind – to fit into a new dress, look 'buff' on the beach holiday or look good in upcoming wedding photos.

This intense campaign is normally based around a new diet with an emphasis on consuming fewer calories (assuming that weight-loss is a goal), perhaps accompanied by an exercise routine of some sort, frequently featuring the 'regular' use of a gym with its array of resistance and cardio machines.

Sometimes, through following a regime like this the stated goals can indeed be met (e.g. lose 9 pounds of fat by March); more often, however, they're not. More likely, the trainee strays from the path they've set themselves and fail to see the programme through to the end.

Whether or not these goals are met, the usual pattern is that after a certain amount of time our once-keen dieter and exerciser returns to their previous habits. Sooner rather than later, the individual finds themselves back in the condition they were in before they started their programme:

Any pounds that *were* lost are quickly regained and, more often than not, a few more pounds are added to take the belt out one more hole! Any benefits of all the hardship are quickly buried beneath a new malaise of inactivity. The individual then feels the shame of having failed to reach their goals.

We've all been there right?

They will get over their failure in time and – sooner or later – will begin another project of self-improvement based on the deluded hope that they can summon higher levels of will power this time round, or that a little tweaking to their programme will make all the difference.

Remember what Einstein said about *continuing to do the same thing but expecting different results*? I'd like to suggest that there is a third way; a third option that avoids the folly of the two most common approaches to fitness and health.

Instinctive Fitness – The Third Way

OK, I'm going to hold my hands up here and admit you *are* going to have to make some changes to your life. I'm not offering a magical silver bullet that will banish the pounds, build the muscle and present you with greater health for free. But IF is not just another fad regime, instead it is a philosophy that offers the most natural way of getting in to and *maintaining* a great level of fitness.

I'm not going to mislead you and claim there is no effort needed here to get started – there is. You're probably going to have to roll your sleeves up for the first 30 days, stick to the rules like glue and *then* let the results speak for themselves.

The biggest carrot I can offer you is that if you choose to take the challenge for just 30 days you will never *want* to go back to your old habits. It will also provide the most compelling evidence that everything I'm about to suggest will get your body back how mother nature intended, given a bit longer on the programme.

A natural fitness

By eating plenty of genuinely satisfying food and by making exercise easier and more fun than you've probably ever known, and refusing to stress and strain over it all, fitness and health *can* be effortlessly maintained. Once the first 30 days are out of the way, it's actually an easier habit to maintain than returning to the alternative 'time bomb' or the martyr's way of living.

I believe that getting in shape – and staying in shape – shouldn't involve Herculean amounts of effort or the will power of Ghandi. The approach to take is one of sustainable long-term change. The basic rule is:

Make Small, Comfortable Changes You Can Keep Up Forever!

Therefore, what I'm proposing is neither a diet (which has a ring of the temporary about it right from the outset) nor a programme of frantic activity with a beginning and an end. Instead, IF is an immensely enjoyable and rewarding **Lifestyle!**

*It's about making minor lifestyle changes that are so painless, so easy to follow, so rewarding and offer such life enhancing results that it's easy to keep them up **forever**.*

That isn't to say that either you or I won't ever overindulge ourselves again, as we surely will; but the difference when keeping yourself fit *Instinctively* is that you'll feel great when you do and worse when you don't, and if you do succumb to temptation you'll actually *look forward* to getting back on track straight away.

Nobody is suggesting that the transition will be really, really easy. However, once the switch has been made, there's little effort needed to sustain the moment, and little incentive to turn back the clock to old habits. You will have developed a new instinct that should see you good for the rest of your life.

Role Models

I believe it can be helpful to develop some new models of fitness to inspire us and realign us with our best intentions.

To do this, I'm not going to suggest any famous Austrian Bodybuilders (either in their prime or their embarrassing flabby, coronary-challenged present), or media personalities such Brad Pitt or Jenifer Aniston whom people admire for their beautifully presented bodies. This is simply because:

Instinctive Fitness shouldn't all be all about **what you look like.**

I'd like to offer you some alternative role models who offer a beauty and depth greater than your average catwalk model or boy band member. People with not only an innate *physical* strength, but a strength of character that makes them the embodiment of that most primitive and glorious human spirit.

1. Gymnasts and Decathletes/Heptathletes

These really can be considered among the king of modern athletes.

Pro: an incredible bodyweight-to-strength ratio, speed, endurance, flexibility, co-ordination, balance, focus and concentration, great agility and low body-fat; also, there's very little 'chronic cardio' in their programme.

Con: They work out for many exhausting hours a day; the female gymnasts often have poor posture from having to pose with a backward leaning spine on completing difficult landings; too many females eat poorly (and like mice) in order to keep their small stature and light-weight frames.

2. Warriors

These can bring to mind whatever image is most powerful for you. Think of greatest warriors from any time or place.

Pro: Strength, endurance, speed, spontaneity of movement, power, awareness, balance, patience, ability to adapt.

Con: Not all warriors are as mobile, flexible and injury resistant as they should be. A lesser breed depends too heavily on sheer strength rather than quality and speed of movement. Soldiers in marine and infantry regiments suffer from repetitive stress injuries far too commonly. For women, the image of the warrior queen or that of the Amazonian women can be a helpful one.

3. The Caveman or Cavewoman (My favourite, of course!)

Pro: Resilient, Strong, stamina-filled, 100% natural human movement patterns, health, explosive speed, awareness of nature, low-body fat, high body-to-weight ratio.

Con: Might have been short of nutrients during very hard times.

If it helps to hold one of these models in your mind, then please do so – maybe even Google a few images to refer to. All manifest the sort of all-round fitness and health that I have been lionising in this book so far.

Alternatively, you might choose a modern individual to inspire you. You might choose **Bruce Lee**, who had one leg-shorter than the other, was badly short-sighted, bullied as a child, shorter than average height, of mixed race, and had damaged his back so badly he was told he'd never kick again. However, none of this stopped him becoming the greatest martial artist ever and the first ever Asian Hollywood star.

Or you might choose **Jack LaLanne**, the US fitness guru who, aged 70, handcuffed, shackled, and fighting strong winds and currents, swam 1 mile towing 70 rowboats, one containing several guests, from the Queen's Way Bridge in the Long Beach Harbour to the *Queen Mary.*[1]

You could look into the lifestyle of **Professor Art de Vany**, who (on a Paleo diet) trains by pushing and pulling his Range Rover up and down his drive. Art is 70 years old and has less than 8% body fat (which is about the same as a professional bodybuilder!).

Or, more recently and closer to home, consider the achievements of **Eddie Izzard** who ran around the perimeter of the UK in 7 weeks in 2009 in back-to-back marathons, or **David Walliams** who swam the length of the Thames in 2010. Both of these comedians (what is it about comedians?) were fairly sedentary until they put their minds to their new challenges. Of course I can't really recommend Izzard's extreme endurance feats, but I can't help admiring his courage and total dedication to the task.

Regardless of whether any of these particular models inspire you, I want you to see if you can conceptualise the sort of fitness and health you might gain by considering **performance**.

Here are a few questions for you to consider. For most of these questions, if the answer is a no, then an imperative should have been set-up – turn this to a yes!

Real World Fitness Test

a) *Could you jump a 5 foot ditch (perhaps even from standing)?*

b) *Could you still climb a tree to rescue an animal or stuck child, or perhaps evade an animal?*

c) *Could you hurdle a garden gate if the hinge is stuck?*

d) *Could you carry an adult out of a burning building?*

e) *Could you get to the top floor of a 6-storey building, taking the steps at a run, two at a time?*

f) *Could you run for a bus at 90% of the top speed you have ever reached in your whole life?*

g) *Could you drag a heavy fallen branch off the road?*

If you find yourself saying: "Yeah, right – at my age!" then you've bought into the prevailing myth of *degeneration with time*. I know individuals in their 70s who can do all of these things.

These questions all emphasise the ability to achieve real ends, the abilities that make our lives greater for their presence, and those abilities that, in times of peril, will change people's lives forever. This, to my mind, is **real fitness, and it is clearly a very different prospect than the mere LOOK of fitness.**

Bearing these kinds of endeavour in mind will keep the coming challenges real. Maybe you'll never quite manage all of these achievements; however, there's accomplishment in every inch you move in this direction, and there's the satisfaction of knowing your ambitions are real.

All-round health

Another area I would like to be hyper-specific about is that of health. Having spoken about the topic in general, I need to make it clear that we can go beyond subjective personal assessments such as:

- *Immunity ('Oh I haven't been ill for years y'know')*
- *Energy ('I just feel so much perkier these days')*
- *Anti-ageing ('Bet you thought I was in my 30s?')*
- *Absence of pain ('Nothing hurts!')*
- *Mental health ('I'm coming down off the bridge now!')*

These are, of course, each a fine 'result' – but they are impossible to quantify.

Instead I want to point you towards very clear markers of health that professionals now consistently rely on for a more scientific picture of the body's true resilience.

These markers include:

- *resting heart-rate*
- *blood-sugar levels*
- *blood pressure*
- *body fat percentage, (or hip to waist ratio)*
- *bone density*
- *hormonal balance*
- *lipid level.*

Only by working closer with doctors are we ever going to persuade the general public and the wider medical community that there is another option on the table. With specific data, we can demonstrate the universal application of the sort of approach I'm advocating.

So get yourself along to your GP and get a check-up to make sure you're fit enough to face the coming challenge – which will also give you a baseline against which to measure future progress.

The proof of the pudding...

So far there is massive anecdotal evidence for the efficacy of the ideas I'm putting forward; there is also a logical, anthropological reasoning, and well-documented but ultimately scattered research to back it all up. What there isn't enough of at the moment is consensus of opinion and mainstream recognition.

By contacting your doctor and getting as many relevant tests done as possible, you will reinforce your awareness of your own success and demonstrate the soundness of these principles to the wider community.

"I have the body of an eighteen year old.
I keep it in the fridge."

Spike Milligan

Chapter Key points:

- *There's a third way that stands apart from harmful sedentary habits and the profitless way many people spend their time trying to reach their fitness goals.*

- *It works with our own nature, our Stone Age bodies, and our unaltered genetic blueprint to bypass our too often fragile willpower.*

- *Good models for fitness are gymnasts, warriors and pre-historic cave-dwellers.*

- *Real world tests and challenges are better than counting repetitions.*

- *You only need to do 3 things well: "Move Well, Eat Well, Live Well".*

References:

1. Wikipedia (2012) Jack LaLanne [Online] Available at: http://en.wikipedia.org/wiki/Jack_LaLanne

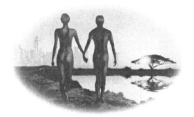

CHAPTER EIGHT

Natural Movement

*"We see in order to move;
we move in order to see"*

William Gibson

Running, jumping, climbing, skipping? So what? Why should any of us move about too much when we simply don't need to anymore - with cars, buses, trains, escalators, TV remote controls and even stair lifts increasingly happy to take the strain?

So let's start right from the beginning with a dumb question:

"Why do we need to move?"

Try to give the simplest all-encompassing answer to this question. The best I've come up with is

"...because movement IS life."

If we are unsure of something's status as a living thing, the first thing we look for is movement. The more self-directed movement we see in a creature (or plant), the more we can be sure it is indeed alive. Movement, whether we are talking about the contraction of capillaries squeezing blood around our bodies or the twitching of a suspiciously still caterpillar's leg, is the stuff of life. To a very real extent, the amount of life left in a thing can be measured by its capacity to move.

As humans, once we start to 'slow down' or to 'take things easy' (physically speaking), we begin an inevitable slow degradation in physical ability, and ultimately the foreshortening of life begins.

"So many older people, they just sit around all day long and they don't get any exercise. Their muscles atrophy, and they lose their strength, their energy and vitality by inactivity."

Jack LaLanne

Humans engage in many different types of movement. Some of these movement are **involuntary** (such as the beating of your heart, or the inhalation of air); some are *voluntary* (skipping down the road with joy, maybe); some are of *necessity* (climbing the stairs or carrying groceries); some are for *pleasure* (dancing on a Saturday night); and some are a matter of pure *self-discipline* (most workout programmes). Perhaps a final category is *resistance of movement* (this includes, but is not limited to, the largely subconscious fight against gravity that good balance and posture involves).

If movement is life, then looking *to improve the quantity and quality of all of our movement* has to be the cornerstone of any approach to a better and longer time spent on Earth.

Earlier in the book we looked at the idea that what much of what plagues modern humans comes out of a mismatch between their modern environment (and modern sedentary habits) and the confused instincts of the stone-age body we all inhabit.

Our first step, therefore, should be to see *where* we are out of step.

Ancient Movements

In past millennia, we would have *had* to move a whole lot more. There was greater need for both sustained, low-effort movements (for example, walking from one hunting ground to another) and the sort of explosive movements necessary to either catch prey or avoid becoming it. I would like to describe what could have been a typical day in the life of our hunter-gatherer ancestors before they shackled themselves to the field and the hoe.

For ease of exposition, I did consider calling the main character of my narrative 'Ugg' or something similarly primitive sounding; however, to do so would be to fall into the trap of stereotyping and trivialising the intelligence of this man and his abilities. In many ways he is our equal (arguably even superior). He communicates well, plans ahead, makes use of technology and takes care of his family in a world with no 'catch net'.

In some ways, he *is* a little more limited than humans today. His knowledge of science is scant (although he does understand fire!), he only knows one way of life, and he is prone to superstition.

In another sense though, he really is our superior. He's incredibly capable physically; he carries very little fat; he's very strong and resilient; is hyper-aware of his environment and is constantly alert to danger. He is also more relaxed and suffers no long-term stress; his values are uncontaminated by the conflicting messages of popular culture; and he is always more concerned with caring for his family and their survival than he is about appearances and keeping up with the Joneses in the next cave along.

Oh, he also has a larger brain than us! According to Matt Ridely, author of *The Agile Gene*, a human living 50,000 years ago had a brain of about 1,500cl compared with today's grain-based brain of 1,250cl.

For these reasons, I shan't patronise him: I shall call him Maerk. The spelling change is just enough to remind us that he does have some differences from us (despite the fact that after a shave, a spruce up and some modern clothes, he would be unlikely to stand out from anyone else on a crowded street).

I want my simple account of Maerk's day to give an idea of how he spends his time. I want you to consider his day by looking at the movements he makes and the exertion they involve.

Maerk's life was full of natural obstacles and challenges that needed to be overcome every day, but fortunately both the wisdom handed down to him by his parents and millions of years of evolution had furnished him with a set of instincts and responses so he and his family could react quickly, decisively and powerfully to any environmental challenge.

Maerk awakens with the sun, as he does every day; earlier in the summer and later in the winter. He rises from his bed fully refreshed from a great night's sleep. He feels instantly energised as well as limber and flexible. Standing tall, straight and strong he sniffs the air and scans the distant horizon to get a feel for the coming day. He must access fresh water, so emerging from his make-shift dwelling he jogs with effortless fluid movements and gentle pace the two hundred yards across the flood plain in little time. (It's still pretty cold at this time in the morning so the jog helps keep him warm).

Filling a skin bottle full of fresh water, he returns with a lightness of foot over the uneven ground to find his wife and child are now also up and preparing items for today's trip. The natural ebb and flow of life is forcing them to walk into the next valley as local game has been scarce for the last couple of days. This is the most likely way they will find the natural resources they had not managed to find nearby lately.

Today, breakfast isn't an option. Some days they have a ready supply of nuts and berries or perhaps left-overs from the previous night's feast. Having nothing to eat, however, is not a particularly big issue for Maerk and his family, as missing a meal or two – although not something they would choose – does happen from time to time.

A low-carbohydrate diet means that they are not so utterly dependent as we are today on a constant supply of glucose to keep feelings of hunger at bay. Their primary energy systems run on fat; both the fat stored on their own bodies and fats they consume in their diet - and they had plenty of that in last night's meal. Should there be a prolonged shortage of fuel, their body will immediately dip into their own constantly turning over fat reserves to keep energy levels constant.

For most of the year Maerk and his family carry very little excess fat on their lithe, well-proportioned frames. When they do find themselves carrying a little extra, they are pleased and feel easier. They know it is insurance against times of lower calorific supply and will hold them in good stead during leaner times.

Setting out over the uneven terrain, Maerk and his family easily adapt their gait to the rocky, uneven ground they cross, placing each leather-covered *(or bare) foot down with a balance, nimbleness and variety of position that would be impossible for those of us more familiar with flat concrete and the deadening effect of thick shoes. Although each family member is pretty strong by today's standards, they still have a level of agility, grace and poise that puts modern, muscle-bound gym monsters to shame.*

A scramble across the rocky riverbed leads them to the bank of a small river. Holding hands, and with their child, Arun, placed on Maerk's shoulders, they easily wade through the bracingly cold river against the strong flow. They are only able to avoid the strongest, mid-stream current by pulling themselves up onto the rocks and nimbly jumping between them. Some of the jumps are as big as five feet, but adult and child alike achieve this distance with well-practised safety and confidence. Back in the water, the cold of the river once again hits them and, although they don't know it, their immune systems are given a sudden boost by the 'feel good' endorphins and stimulating hormones their bodies release automatically in response.

They walk on for a few hours, their good pace only interrupted by Maerk's insistence on stopping to climb trees to appease his craving for the sweet 'hit' of the year's first supply of honey. (Honey is pretty much the only really sweet taste they know, with the exceptions of fruit, which itself is sourer than our modern cultivated equivalents.)

Maerk's wife, Jeel, indulges his optimism. She knows it will be weeks yet before honey is available, but Maerk's tooth is sweeter than hers and he cannot wait. All the time Jeel keeps a keen eye on both Arun, practising climbing like dad in a smaller tree nearby, and for potential threats lurking in the immediate environment. She knows that to get lost in reverie or day-dreaming could be a costly mistake in this dangerous territory.

Indeed, crossing the corner of a forest, they walk right into the presence of a buffalo with young calves. They know this is a bad-tempered animal and are unable to defend themselves without the presence of other members of their tribe. Backing off, they are forced to retreat from the forest before sprinting off back the way they have come. They will need to find another route. Although Arun is only ten, he is a seasoned runner, and almost able to keep up with the top speed of both his parents, despite them both being not far short of today's Olympic standard athletes.

This 300 yard dash leaves everyone breathing heavily, partly from the intensity of the sprint and partly from the adrenaline rush of the encounter. But as soon as is safe, they drop the pace to a jog and exchange smiles and accounts of what had just happened. This will not become something to fret or dwell on however; it was just a fact of life. With their high levels of anaerobic fitness, their breathing rates quickly return to comfortable levels again and they continue on their way. Despite their efforts, they feel energised and invigorated, rather than drained.

They know it is possible they may have to run like that again at any moment, so they try to ensure they take it easy while they can. Arun breaks this rule, of course. He runs, plays, skips and chases like any child...

At noon, the day's hottest point, they know to stop to get out of the mid-day sun for a well-deserved rest under the shade of a willow by a meander in the river (after all they have walked for a couple of hours already today). They've been snacking on whatever edible berries, nuts and seeds they came across during their walk and, although they are still hoping to catch meat today, they are ready for a rest.

The adults take it in turns to doze in the sun while the other parent teaches Arun how to catch fish with his hands. With perseverance and not a few missed opportunities there is much laughter and rejoicing when Arun catches the first fish of his young life, which is quickly added to other items the family have collected to cook later.

Arriving at their destination after their break, they set about acclimatising and tuning in to their new environment. This forest has not been populated by humans for a while and is abundant in wildlife – just as Maerk had predicted. It isn't long before they manage to bag a small monkey with a skilful throw of the spear, and Arun is entrusted with the task of carrying the carcass on top of all the other goodies he has foraged along the way. It's not light for him, but he isn't new to this sort of challenge.

Finally, at about 1.30pm, they find what they've been hoping for: a wild pig. Jeel and Arun work together to herd the pig into a trap. This involves crawling around on the forest floor in order to avoid being observed, before jumping to their feet and chasing the creature through the trees.

With brutal precision and speed the pig is driven right onto the point of Maerk's spear, and he kills it with a quick twist.

Now happy and furnished with the wealth of natural provisions they came for, they need to get to high ground for its added security. They retrace their steps back out of the valley, clambering back up the steep sides of the canyon towards the plateau where they had strategically camped. The return journey is quicker as there is less emphasis on checking for animal tracks and possible food sources, but they are slowed a little by the weight of the heavy pig, which must be borne between the two adults.

Back at the camp, Jeel butchers the pig carefully; they have both been taught by elders that no part of the beast must be wasted. (Eating the whole animal, including the organs, ensures that they miss no vital nutrients that their bodies need, even when plants are scarce in the winter.) She adds some small lean natural root vegetables that she found growing nearby after a brief forage.

Maerk knows that it will be soon be dark and the dinner needs cooking. He finds a large fallen branch a few hundred yards away, and, assisted by Arun, drags it back to the camp. He then proceeds to chop this branch with a stone axe into smaller logs suitable for the fire that they will soon be squatting around while their generous supper cooks.

It has been a tough physical day by any modern standard. The family has walked, climbed, lunged, sprinted, crawled, thrown, lifted, pulled, chopped, dragged, jumped, swam, squatted, carried... pretty much every human movement you can think of, but they've also not stressed about their lot, and found time for fun and relaxation too. They've done everything at a sustainable pace, rather than risking exhaustion, and now have a feeling of quiet satisfaction from having survived another day.

In fact they only pushed themselves to their limits once (for about a minute when running away from the buffalo), but they were active in a low-key way for most of the day. Even just minutes after the encounter with the buffalo their bodies' stress chemicals, which for a brief time had flooded into their bloodstream to provide them with extra energy, had quickly returned back to their normal low levels.

As they settle down for another dark night with no illumination other than the fire embers and the glowing stars, they have nothing on their minds to disturb their rest: no to-do lists, no business meeting to prepare for and no mortgage payments to worry about.

The next few days will undoubtedly be easier. Their giant pig will supply them with easy access to food for some time and the daytime will bring an opportunity to join up with the other families to joke, laugh and perhaps enjoy some dancing.

A fateful contrast

This is the life of Maerk and his family. What's more it's roughly representative of human life on earth for 98% of the time we have had any sort of tenure here on this planet.

Please take a moment, if you haven't already, to consider your own day. What demands does it generally place upon you? What physical exercise do you get? For many people, in terms of movement; it goes something like this:

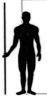

"Rise, walk a few steps, descend stairs, sit, eat, walk a few steps, five breaths of fresh air, drive, walk a few steps, sit, sit, eat, sit, sit, walk a few steps, drive, walk a few steps, take 5 breaths of fresh air, eat, sit, ascend stairs, sleep"

Even if you have a 40-minute period dedicated to exercise, I bet it was either a plod on a treadmill or a self-inflicted 'beasting'! Can you see how different it is to Maerk's family's experience of life. Their day *was* movement – continual movement interspersed with periods of relaxation. Our days, by contrast, are filled with large quantities of sitting, tiny amounts of movement and regular carb-filled meals. When we look at it like this, it really isn't hard to see how so many of us have gone wrong.

And what stresses does your average day inflict upon you? What mental pressures are you under, what timetable do you have to work to? What do you worry about 24 hours a day, 7 days a week? And finally, when was the last time your body was flooded with adrenalin for 'fight or flight' and you knew you were truly alive?

My hypothesis is this: for every little change you can make that takes your experience of life a little closer to a life like Maerk's, you will be healthier and the happier for it.

Please notice that I said *'like'* Maerk's world. I am not suggesting some sort of ancient history re-enactment activity; that you return to the woods, become a hunter-gatherer, throw away your food blender, or try hunting wild pig in Nottingham Forest.

However, there are elements of your life that you *can* change to be more like Maerk's that will serve your hard wired instincts, and in aggregate, improve your life beyond measure.

In the rest of this chapter I will outline how you can easily change your movement habits and patterns to become more 'Maerk-like'. In other words:

- *more energy*
- *lower body fat*
- *greater muscle mass*
- *more endurance*
- *better balance*
- *more speed*
- *greater range of movement and flexibility*

- *better immunity to illness*
- *fewer signs of ageing*
- *less stress*
- *better moods*
- *less dependency on drugs*
- *lowered risk of diabetes*

A big claim I know!

What is 'caveman fit'?

If you really want to get into a 'caveman fit' shape, you're going to need to carry out movements which featured heavily in Maerk's day; they will need to feature prominently in *your* programme if you are to achieve the same sort of all-round fitness that he and his family possessed.

Maerk's average day was made up like this:

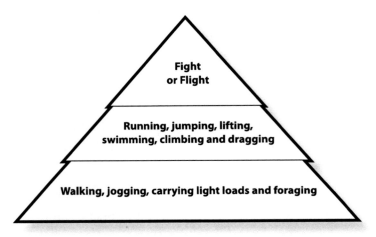

So, in short, he wasn't banging away doing the same type of movement every time he was active. All round fitness shouldn't be about isolating one body part and hitting it intensely to get a single aesthetic result. Your overall vitality is only ever as strong as your weakest link.

Which brings us nicely onto the IF model of exercise.

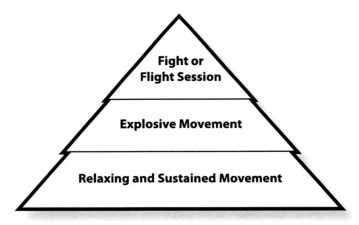

This is the model of exercise that we think Maerk would have recognised and approved. We can use this to replicate the everyday demands placed on his body.

Of course there are other categories to be considered when talking about physical fitness.

Put very broadly, these alternative, more mainstream, categories are:

1. **Maximum strength**
2. **Posture, flexibility and poise (all related)**
3. **Speed**
4. **Agility**
5. **Balance**

Let's look at each in turn

Maximum Strength:

Maximum Strength is anyone's maximum instant capacity to move a heavy weight, and the amount you can lift off the ground is a very basic measure of 'maximum strength'. Now think back on Maerk's day, as well as your own. How many times are you called upon to exert your maximum capacity in an instant? Most likely, never at all – and the same is true for Maerk.

Now and again Maerk might have dragged a branch or lifted an animal that was at the absolute edge of his maximum strength, but generally he would work safely within his full capacity. The exception to this was, of course, when he dragged the heavy fallen branch back to the camp. So, in fact, with some further thought, we've established that maximum strength work (category one) isn't much of a day-to-day feature of Maerk's life, so it doesn't need to play a huge role in yours, unless you especially want it to.

(You don't need to become an Olympic lifter. Phew!)

Posture, flexibility and poise

This is something that Meark would never have consciously worked at – but then he never had to. He retained good posture and the flexibility that comes with that throughout his life merely by engaging in natural movement every day.

Speed, Agility and Balance

These are co-ordination issues and once you start to exercise and move in a more natural way, the Instinctive Fitness model delivers fantastic speed, agility and balance results without needing to practice these qualities in isolation.

For most of us interested in our health and pursuing a superior body, these last three come naturally when following a more natural or 'functional' fitness plan. When designing a programme for an individual client I might include some aspects of these elements but, for the most part, homing in on the other categories promotes all-round performance while bringing out these other qualities without further specific attention.

Let's focus on what *is* important

Let's tune in to these 3 key areas that make up the pillars of IF:

- *Fight or Flight Sessions*
- *Explosive Movement*
- *Relaxed and Sustained Movement*

Here we are focusing right in on the essential components of a pure thoroughbred human. Trust me, if you can get *these* qualities nailed down, you will be fitter than pretty much everybody you know. You'll be capable of turning your new found natural fitness abilities to whatever the situation requires – whether that be responding to an emergency or simply leaving every other father for dead in the Fathers' Race at your kid's school.

Also, while I'm not overly concerned with appearance, you'll also end up looking fairly 'ripped', as the expression goes. You'll never look like Stallone or Schwarzenegger used to, but you've probably got the potential to look a bit like Henry Cavill in 'Immortals' or Hilary Swank in 'Million Dollar Baby'.

If that sounds ridiculous, then remember that I am not suggesting that this sort of change happens overnight. If you are woefully out of shape (I'm thinking – to keep the Hollywood theme going – of the "Nutty Professor" look), then it might take a year or two.

Even if you don't quite reach these dizzy aesthetic heights (I am not denying differing genetic potentials), if you stick with the right programme you will end up toned, wiry, nimble, fleet-of-foot, powerful for your weight, super-charged with energy and with a whole new vigour. *You do need to combine this, however, with the eating patterns outlined in the next chapter if you are to get even half-way towards these ideals.*

Let's look at these three aspects in turn.

Explosive Movement

In Instinctive Fitness we call any short, sharp, high intensity movement an **'Explosive Movement'.** These are not to be confused with your tri-weekly run to exhaustion on your gym's cross-trainer!

Explosive Movement is your body's ability to apply a comparatively high amount of force and to continue to do so over a restricted period of time. Any exertion that extends over this time period results in rapidly getting out of breath, pain and massive performance loss because you'll be using your **anaerobic pathway.**

Anaerobic What??!! Anaerobic' means 'without oxygen', and when exercising like a demon you'll inevitably very soon notice fatigue and pain in the muscles through lactic acid build up and a quick deterioration in movement quality.

> Anaerobic exercise is a short, high intensity effort with which your heart and lungs cannot (in the long term) keep up. So in effect, once you are working hard enough to go anaerobic you're living on borrowed time and exhaustion is not too far away.

Maerk was in this zone when he was jumping between rocks, climbing trees, running from animals with explosive acceleration and cutting up fallen branches. He was totally incapable of keeping up any of these feats for an *extended* period of time, so didn't even try – but he *is* capable of pursuing these activities with ease for a constrained period without immediate fatigue or discomfort.

If *you* are easily fatigued by running fifty yards for a bus, climbing three flights of stairs, using a foot pump, carrying grocery bags, or walking up steep hills, Explosive Movement is an area that might need some serious attention. This was the area of fitness that was so badly missing in my gardener client Lee's programme.

Getting into the Explosive Movement Zone

The good news is that this sort of fitness improves quite quickly when you approach it in the right way. Twenty minutes or so of a few brief exertions, two or three times a week, will pay noticeable dividends within just a couple of weeks. (You might not lose much weight in this time, but you will quickly start to avoid fatigue when previously it would have had you red-faced and puffing like an embarrassed, elderly steam-train.)

The effect of this comparatively high intensity training is to develop your body's ability to supply enough oxygen and glucose to the muscles fast enough. In doing so, you will develop additional strength in those muscles. Sometimes with this type of training, muscles can grow larger, although this depends on many other factors, especially nutrition. It is more useful as an aid to weight-loss than it is a genuine muscle-building programme.

Don't get me wrong, you WILL get considerably stronger, and your physical capacity will grow, but if you measure your biceps every morning you will probably be disappointed; it would be better instead to measure your waistline every week or so.

At this point, having decided that the benefits of this sort of training are definitely for you, you have a few different choices when it comes to implementation.

Build this sort of movement into your day with **Heavy Resistance Tasks**

or

Commit to an **Explosive Movement Session** *2 or 3 times a week.*

Building heavy resistance tasks into your day

Ideally you would simply do tasks that require this sort of sustained effort. Even more ideally, they would require no time input at all as they'd be tasks that actually *needed* doing anyway. Examples of this would be chopping logs for a fire with an axe, raking up leaves, digging a hole, carrying bricks in a wheel barrow, using a sledge hammer, moving furniture and sawing branches into logs – but whatever you do, do it with some vigour!

If you are less fit, simply vacuuming the house, dusting, painting and other household chores will help. If you're a bit fitter, these won't challenge you so much but can still be counted towards your Relaxing and Sustained activities for the week.

Including this sort of activity in your week on a number of occasions will get you reasonably fit and strong. Over time, you can build considerable strength, technique and some reasonable cardiac capacity.

Of course, the advantages of this approach are that if the tasks need doing anyway, in effect, it doesn't take any time at all; and all of these activities involve authentic human movement patterns (unlike the ab-curl machine at the gym which will only speed up your transformation into a hunchback).

A disadvantage of relying solely on this approach is that your heart and cardiovascular system won't be worked quite as well as it would be with a more formal workout discussed later. You would only need to add something like simple sprints once a week to iron out this omission however.

Who knows? All this log chopping and carrying may have you fancying going the whole hog: moving to a log cabin, growing your own vegetables, raising your own grass-fed livestock, hunting for edible fauna in the woods, living entirely off your own labours... Okay, well maybe not; but somebody might?

Option two: Commit to 2 or 3 Explosive Movement sessions a week.

This is going to be a good option for many of you who live a life of relative ease and can't easily manufacture the excuse to add new activities of the sort listed above to your day. This can be very simple if you wish it. You could even do an identical routine each day, but ideally you would add some variation to maintain interest and encourage progression.

Here are the basic principles:

- *Arrange your exercises as a circuit, one exercise followed by the next one. (Don't use sets. For our purposes that would be a waste of time)*

- *Rest as little as you can between exercises*

- *Choose exercises which exercise large groups of muscles or the whole body in one go.*

- *When one area of the body gets a rest, hit that area with the next exercise*

- *Take a rest between circuits if your breathing has become uncomfortably laboured*

- *Do each exercise for a given amount of time (or until it becomes uncomfortable – whichever happens sooner)*

Here's an example of Richard's (a client of mine) basic routine. It contains only simple, natural movements which don't leave any muscle group unworked. (You could argue that any other routine is just a fancy variant of this one.) Richard is 39 and wasn't previously inactive, but when he's honest he admits he hasn't done a press-up since school.

The only equipment needed for this routine is a timer and something to pull-up on (the pull up is an essential move). The overhead press you can do with anything at all that you consider 'quite' heavy. Even a chair would work. The whole body is worked out fully: muscles, heart, and lungs. The body enjoys a kick of adrenaline and endorphins are released into it that the mind revels in. At the end of the workout Richard feels more vital, more alive, and ready to go off and ***do*** things; he is not thinking about where to lie down and die. This is not because he is super-fit; Richard just knows when to stop and how to respect his body's limits.

Richard's Explosive Movement Workout

1. Press-ups *(30 secs) [chest, shoulders, arms]*

2. Squats *(30 secs) [legs]*

3. Pull-ups *(30 secs) [biceps and back]*

4. Overhead press *(30 secs) [chest, shoulders and arms]*

5. Lunges *(30 secs) [legs]*

6. Plank *(30 secs) [core muscles]*

Rest for 1 minute - REPEAT 3 TIMES

Too hard?

1. Press-ups – do them from your knees instead of your toes, or against a wall.

2. Squats – only do the first 1/3 of a squat before ascending.

3. Pull-up – jump up to top position and then slow your descent. Use a Theraband around your legs tied to the bar to make it even easier.

4. Overhead press – use a light weight only, like two bricks.

5. Lunges – take smaller lunges forward.

6. Plank – do them from your knees instead of your feet.

Too easy?

1. Press-up – raise one foot, keep hands narrow and level with low ribs.

2. Squats – go all the way down or hold an object as you squat.

3. Pull-ups – use a super wide grip.

4. Overhead press – use something heavier.

5. Lunges – hold a weight in each hand.

6. Plank – lift a foot, or an arm and the opposite foot.

On the IF website at www.instinctive-fitness.com there are many video/ pictures showing many Explosive Movement exercises – even for those who might initially struggle to get started

As you can see, there is no gap between exercises; they run one into another. Richard has allowed himself 30 seconds for each exercise and has 6 exercises in his circuit. At the end of each circuit he will rest for one minute. This means that his routine will last exactly 12 minutes. (Richard has never tried telling me he can't find 12 minutes in his day.) I say 'exactly' because, if he feels that he will struggle to continue any exercise for the whole 30 seconds without a feeling of unpleasant fatigue, he will rest until the end of that 30 second period before commencing the next exercise.

It must not hurt!!

If this isn't your experience of this sort of exercise – you're doing it wrong! Like Maerk, *you don't need to push yourself beyond the natural boundaries that your body lays down for you either.* Your body knows how much exercise it needs to progress and will try to protect you from doing more than you need (which would delay recovery and diminish health) by reducing your enjoyment of the experience.

When this happens, one part of the mind remembers the experience and finds all sorts of excuses not to participate in this sort of ritual ever again. This is when it becomes difficult to establish the motivation to workout. When the mind behaves like this, it is throwing the baby out with the bath water, but you have spent time conditioning it to believe that exercise must be effortful and uncomfortable – so you can hardly blame it for adding two and two in this way.

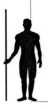

A challenge

If you want a real challenge, instead of seeing how knackered you can feel at the end of a session, see if you can complete a workout (or just one circuit) while only breathing deeply through your nose. With practice this is possible and it ensures that you never leave the boundaries within which your body will prosper, enjoy and thank you for.

"Exercise is labour without weariness."

Samuel Johnson

This session takes just 12 minutes – and, repeated a few times a week, could revolutionise what you are capable of in a matter of half-a-dozen weeks. Over the course of years, it could mean the difference between having to watch your grandchildren play from the deckchair or chasing them around the garden.

Mix it up – Make it fun!

As you get better with Richard's simple routine, there will come a time when you need to change this in order to continue reaping the benefits. Here's what to do:

- *Change some of the exercises*
  (perhaps adds some free weights)

- *Add another circuit*
  (especially if you started with less than 3 circuits)

- *Add one or two additional exercises on the end of the circuit*

- *Increase the 30 seconds to 45 seconds or a minute*

- *Cut out the minute's rest between circuits*

- *Add a light jog (30 seconds or so) between each exercise.*

Perhaps alternate between making changes that make your routine longer, and those that make it more intense. Following my dictum of "it doesn't have to hurt", remember that if you are "scheduled" to complete a session but you feel under the weather or poorly-recovered from a previous session, just rest that day and think about restarting the routine when you can.

> If your body needs rest, it'll let you know. There's no need for heroics. Leave your 'whatever-it-takes' Rambo mentality for real emergencies!

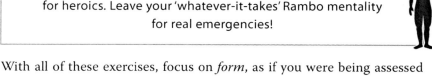

With all of these exercises, focus on *form*, as if you were being assessed for grace rather than strength endurance. Don't kick yourself if you don't do each movement well yet. Treat each movement as *practice*, instead of just a task or exercise.

Fight or Flight Sessions

If you perform the above exercises regularly or organise your life so that plenty of resistance tasks are built into it, you will already be on the way to improving your aerobic capacity (that is, the ability of the heart and lungs to provide your muscles with the oxygen and fuel that they require).

However, if you think back to the description of Maerk's day, there was an event which, in terms of effort, stood out high and dry above the others: the mad dash away from the buffalo herd. Now this sort of event might have happened once or twice a week, and some weeks not at all. However, Maerk never went very long without pushing himself *flat out*, albeit for only a very short amount of time.

This is the point that most people miss when implementing training programmes, so it's actually the biggest secret there is. Most people struggle to get the results that they want because their routine is very predictable and they never push the dial up to ten. Routine training produces routine results... nothing special at all. The problem is that much of their training occupies what I call **'the middle ground to Nowheresville'.**

Middle ground to Nowheresville

Trainees typically push themselves 'quite hard', 'quite a lot'. They do the same thing each week but they either get progressively tired over time (without enough recovery time) or they progress little as their sessions never raise the bar of their maximal efforts. This is what I used to do before I saw the light and it's a recipe for failure as my belly would attest. Remember that as humans it's one of our ten hard-wired instincts to be as lazy as possible, except when a sudden, dire, adrenalin situation occurs. Therefore we would have walked to our destinations in an unhurried fashion, and only jogged or sprinted very occasionally when the situation demanded it.

Go to a running club if you're unconvinced. You won't see much lean muscle mass here (a key marker of rude health). Instead you'll see surprisingly chubby people whose fat tissue has managed to survive all those miles, people with emaciated frames (the beanpoles), or people who have both issues going on (the 'skinny-fat'). You won't see anyone who looks like a sprinter, with noticeably defined muscle, spontaneous power and low body-fat.

This is why I recommend you keep your training easy, even when you're doing explosive movement sessions or working around the house. Don't grind yourself into the ground over the course of weeks.

> All you'll achieve by flogging yourself is to add a lot of stress to your life, and probably quite a lot of muscle wastage.

It's ironic that the marathon event was inspired by the fortunes of its first runner, the Greek Pheidippides, who collapsed and died after completing his feat of endurance. This is an event that people now take up for 'health reasons' and yet the evidence suggests quite the opposite. Regular distance racers suffer depressed immune systems and enjoy a low level of health.

A recent study from the University of Melbourne showed that high-effort endurance activities can lead to scarring of the right ventricle (heart chamber), increasing the risk of health complications. They researchers followed 40 marathon runners and discovered that all of the runners suffered from decreased function of the right ventricle for about a week after the race; in 5 of them the damage to their heart appeared to be permanent.[1]

I don't have anything against the *occasional* long distance event if you fancy taking part, but I'd like to ask you take it easy and not log hundreds of tough miles in preparation for it. In fact, choose an event which is a surprise to your body but doesn't overly tax it. Just enjoy it without worrying about your finishing position. Then allow for plenty of recovery time.

'Distance racing', whether running, cycling, swimming or triathlon, is fine under these conditions, but is entirely optional. I do, however, recommend that once a week you add a bout of the training that really gets me and my clients into amazing shape:

Fight or Flight Training

For this explosively exciting session, all prohibitions about never pushing yourself go out the window. You need to exert **maximal efforts,** as if your life depended on it. (One day it might!) This high intensity approach should leave you feeling exhilarated and re-invigorated. But here's the thing: it should all be done in a very small window of time. Just a few minutes including recovery time is ideal. Because each burst of movement is so short, it's not, psychologically speaking that hard at all. You should be able to recover from these efforts pretty quickly – not because you've held back, but because your efforts didn't last very long.

Our Fight or Flight training approach was inspired by a Japanese researcher called **Nishimura Tabata** who developed what he called the IE1 Protocol. This groundbreaking scientist showed that short, high-intensity bursts of movement (4 mins/day, 4 x a week) could get participants as fit as a control group of trained athletes who logged sessions more than 5 times longer.[2] By the end of the study the former group had a higher VO_2 Max (peak oxygen uptake) and, unlike the control group, has also improved their aerobic capacity.

The benefits are indisputable. HIIT (High Intensity Interval Training) has been shown to improve maximal oxygen consumption and, more recently, to improve insulin action and blood-glucose levels. Michael Mosley presented compellingly new evidence of the advantages of this approach in his 2012 documentary, "The Truth About Exercise" (Horizon, BBC2).

"Your body knows best"

With *Instinctive Fitness* we've taken Tabata's principles one step further by avoiding prescriptive formulas completely and just listening closely to the body. No longer will you need a personal trainer to tell you exactly how long your intervals should be or how much recovery time you are allowed. Instead you'll learn to rely on your own *instinct* for what's best *for you.*

It has been shown that the brain protects the human body by sending messages (in the form of pain) telling it to back away from using its full capacity long before it reaches a dangerous level of exertion. (Dire emergencies are a notable exception to this rule however. When these happen, hormones flood the body allowing one-off 'superhuman' performances from ordinary, untrained individuals that go down in urban legend. People lifting heavy vehicles off crash victims – that sort of thing)

In the IF system of high intensity training, we make use of this natural protective mechanism to greatly reduce the chance of stress, injury and failure. We prefer to listen and respond appropriately to pain rather than to push through it.

The information and feedback your own body provides is 100% accurate, totally natural and offers a safe method for anyone to safely reach their personal optimal training intensity, without any pain and without ever over-stressing themselves.

Here's how we do it: **The IF Fight or Flight Protocol**

a) Choose a method of whole-body movement like running, biking, swimming, free-weight squatting or rowing. (Sprinting on the spot is a great option for beginners or those short on equipment or space.)

b) Perform this movement at your absolute top speed until your body tells you to slow down. This may be in the form of a noticeable performance drop off, or through other physical signs such as painful, laboured breathing, a stitch, other signs of physical discomfort, or just a disinclination to continue.

c) The very moment you feel your body is telling you to back off: BACK OFF! Drop your movements down to a very gentle aerobic level (perhaps 10% of your previous effort).

d) Maintain this level until your body returns to a comfortable, steady level and tells you it's ready to go again.

e) Repeat the cycle until your body is unable to return to a steady, comfortable level. If you're not raring to go flat out again **within 3 minutes**: STOP!

This whole session is likely to be over in just a few minutes! Nevertheless, according to the research on HIIT, this represents a credible and effective method for *anyone*, no matter what their current fitness level or how hectic their schedule, to stave off the spectre of Type-2 diabetes and obesity.

The great thing about this very personal approach is that it grows with you. You will never have to make any decisions about progression, or need to consciously push any harder with each new session. The feedback your own body gives will automatically let you push just that little bit further without trying, minimising the risk of over-exertion or injury.

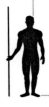

Living on the Edge

If you really need to 'feel the burn' during your fight or flight training, that's fine - but please bear in mind that, from an evolutionary point of view, Maerk would never have dreamed of deliberately leaving himself vulnerable to predators by pushing himself to total exhaustion.

If you absolutely can't help yourself, and really *must* push your personal limits and feel some pain - only do so for a **maximum of 20 - 30 seconds**. Pushed beyond this, future performances will not necessarily be the better, and you are certainly compromising your health and immune system.

Before a session like this you'll probably want to warm up a little first. I will say more about stretching later in the book, but suffice to say that all you really need to do is to practice the movements that you are about to perform in a less intense manner. If you are going to sprint, for example, you might first run 30m, then 50m, then 70m, getting up to a higher speed each time.

If you are coming into this session after hours of sitting down, I would recommend some walking or general movements first, as some muscles can be quite tight and prone to injury if suddenly stressed. If you are totally unfit you should take things steady, running at perhaps only 80% of your top speed for the first few sessions.

This session could all be done in 5-10 minutes (including the warm-up time). If you are aiming to burn fat, then doing this sort of thing on an empty stomach (maybe first thing in the morning) is an amazing short-cut to fat loss!

Do this once or twice a week instead of breakfast and you're onto a secret that has been entirely overlooked by mainstream Conventional Wisdom. If you're not already doing something like this, add it to your programme and watch excess flab melt away and your fitness levels soar.

Benefits of sprinting

Remember when you were a kid and you sprinted around the playground for probably no reason, perhaps chasing a football and a whole host of other games were as natural as reaching for the TV remote is now? Remember the thrill and the excitement of games such as 'kick the can' or even good old fashioned 'chase'?

If, like me a couple of years ago, you haven't run at full pelt for a long, *long* time, and when you did give it bash, it felt awkward and your legs just didn't have the zap in them they used too, you'll like this next section.

Sprinting as hard as you can is perhaps one of life's extreme physical pleasures: the feeling of skimming across the ground with (when done in the spirit of play) a lightness and an agility perhaps long since considered consigned to the history books.

Running for short distances it not only great fun, but has a whole heap of health benefits:

1. *Sprinting reduces body fat and reduces insulin sensitivity. (Ever heard of a fat or diabetic sprinter?)*

2. *Sprinting requires maximal recruitment of muscle, so it targets fast twitch muscle fibres much better than slower training. Fast-twitch fibres are thicker than slow twitch fibres, and it is fast twitch fibres that grow in size when activated by the right training.*

3. *Sprinting naturally increases Human Growth Hormone (HGH). HGH increases muscle mass; thickens and adds flexibility to the skin; enhances the immune system; promotes weight loss through fat redistribution and loss; and increases stamina.*

4. *Sprinting strengthens your cardiovascular system with brief bursts of high intensity. Depending on the recovery time you allow yourself, you can work your cardiovascular system more intensely (short recoveries, Tabata style) or concentrate on power, speed and strength (using longer recoveries).*

5. *Sprint workouts are short and a lot more fun than long, boring cardio workouts.*

Go on, find any old excuse – race your children, kick and chase a ball
– anything you can think of to re-ignite that urge to run you
felt naturally as a child!

Fasted exercise

Conventional wisdom will recommend that you should always fuel up before exercise, and always eat three meals a day – plus snacks! However a moment's thought will make it abundantly clear that we didn't evolve with an entirely consistent calorie supply. Our intake of calories would have been irregular and would have depended on our hunting skill and foraging luck.

Sometimes our ancestors would have gone to bed hungry having tried and failed to find food during the day. Days would often have begun without food, and further 'exercise' would be required again before they were likely to acquire any.

In other words, if you're serious about copying our ancestral lifestyle patterns (and serious about fat-loss and health), when you are hungry you should sometimes choose to exercise instead!

Our health can no longer afford (despite our monetary wealth) for us to eat every single time we are hungry. A little rational thought and a dose of discipline should allow us to overcome this once useful urge to eat whenever we can.

Please note that I am not asking you to reduce your calorie intake over anything more than 12 hours, or to do this day after day as most 'diets' require. This is unnecessary, psychologically tough, and usually backfires.

Few can stick with it - but those who do find that much of their reduced weight is not actually fat loss but the disappearance of lean muscle tissue. Almost all later return to their previous weight or heavier, but at a higher percentage body-fat and a lower percentage of muscle. Don't do it!

All I ask is that you consider – either tactically or for convenience – skipping a meal or two each week. I'll give you details on how to do this in **Chapter 9.**

Review

Let's see what we've got so far:

1. **Explosive Movements**, *or daily resistance tasks such as a fairly easy circuit routine that maintain/build muscle mass and anaerobic capacity*

2. **A 'Fight or Flight' session,** *perhaps on a fasted stomach. (15 minutes, maximum, including warm up – 1 or 2 times a week at the most)*

Finally, we need to address the bottom tier of the IF pyramid

Relaxing and Sustained Movement

Relaxing and sustained movements are essentially a greater quantity of low-level intensity movements. Our ancestors varied between being well rested, and performing a considerable amount of low-key movement. A typical estimate by anthropologists is that they covered 7-12 miles a day. Some days they might not have gone very far at all if food stocks were high, but on other days they might cover as much as the full 12 miles.

In the modern age, many of us will struggle to add this sort of level of time commitment into our day. Luckily it's not really needed. Most of the benefits associated **with low-level aerobic work** can be enjoyed with considerably less time investment. However to be Caveman fit, there is no getting away from doing *some*.

I would suggest that the minimum is **3 to 5 hours a week.** With this I would estimate that you will still accrue 70% of the benefits of being mobile for up to ten times longer. You will certainly avoid the massive risks that have been identified with being completely sedentary!

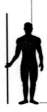

> If you cannot be gently active for 3 hours (out of the 168 in your week), consider that the threat of the sedentary lifestyle has been identified as a continued threat even to those who work out regularly if the rest of their time is divided between being seated and being in bed.

Logging 3-5 hours activity might not be as tough as you think. Firstly, sport counts and it's easy to keep up the time if it's fun. If you play a round or two of golf a week, you're covered. If you play tennis twice a week, you'll be most of the way there (same for squash, badminton, etc). I recommend you play these sports just for fun and don't worry about pushing yourself hard; just enjoy the game and enjoy the process.

If sport isn't your thing then just walk (which is ideal), or cycle or swim very slowly. Maybe take a couple of dance lessons (almost any kind is fine – check out 'Zumba', even if it's just on the Wii). Perhaps get a dog to walk – or borrow one. Or start walking to work. Or walk to the shops and carry your shopping back. (Wow... now that's starting to sound very instinctive, isn't it? Nothing artificial about that at all as long as you can pretend you don't have a car!)

If you've added resistance tasks into your day, they also count towards fulfilling this requirement, as long as your body has recovered from them by the next day.

Anything that gets you moving in any way, shape or form is fine; the point is to try to get at least 3 hours a week where you're not sitting around doing nothing (or working, watching TV or whatever); to the body it's just atrophy after the first 30 minutes.

Other physical training

I don't mean to present my workout programmes listed above as the only way to achieve your goals. I am often asked about the benefits of doing this or that instead. To answer my interrogator I always refer back to our ancient model of fitness and see where any new suggestions align, if at all, with the life of our typical hunter-gatherer.

From the description of Maerk's day earlier, you'll have noticed that everything he does involves moving himself and moving natural objects. I would advise you to try to keep as close to this model as possible. Therefore I would recommend walking over cycling and using your own bodyweight over using any sort of a machine as resistance. Most of the time you should be reconnecting with these natural movement patterns, but an occasional bike or rowing machine workout is harmless enough. I can't stress enough the need for **variety in a programme** to maintain interest and include as many natural movement patterns as possible.

Get some toys

One deviation from body-weight work you might want to make at some point, especially for men, is to make an investment in a barbell, a squat rack, a bench and a set of free weights. This allows a greater degree of strength to be maintained and more muscle growth than using bodyweight alone. However, I would consider this unnecessary for most people until they can attain some basic benchmarks – for men, say 40 press-ups, 12 pull-ups and 50 deep squats. For women, it's half of this.

In a perfect world, all the movements (the squat, press, plank, etc) would be part of a spontaneous expression of part of your life – as it was for Maerk. For clients, I have developed challenges that mirror the same sort that he might have faced. For example, a walk of a good length with some light jogging, followed by quick sprints, finished off with some sort of lifting and carrying activity simulates the pressures of a hunter-gatherer's day more realistically than my basic programme. Such an approach goes beyond the scope of this book, however, and isn't going to be easier or preferable for those looking for a basic, flexible framework with which to begin.

At **www.instinctive-fitness.com** we have material that supports a more creative, spontaneous approach – but it is not guaranteed to get better results than the simple, organised routine that I have already given you.

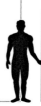

Flexibility

This is a huge topic and I really cannot do it justice here. Where I differ from conventional wisdom is that I believe that specific flexibility and stretching work is only necessary in remedial situations when a specific issue is being addressed. For a martial artist, that could be that they need to improve their hip flexibility so that they can kick to head height. For an injured sportsman, this could be regaining a full range of movement in a joint which has recently suffered some damage.

For people who have postural issues (most of us), very specific dynamic movements can help rebalance resting muscle length of key muscles, alleviate pain, reduce the likelihood of injury and improve performance. Random, general stretching is unlikely to do this.

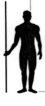

A couple of appointments with a human movement specialist may therefore be a very good investment! They look at your own particular patterns of movement and prescribe a programme for your own, very idiosyncratic body. Check out **www.instinctive-fitness.com** to find a local approved specialist who will help offset all the unnatural movement patterns and positions you have used habitually for years.

Alternatively, if, for example, your pelvis is displaced (as it is with many people) you might see a chiropractor to short-cut your rehabilitation. In a modern world with modern problems, sometimes the answer is a modern solution – again, check out the website for a good chiropractor.

In general, though, if you are active in the widest possible sense and are regularly practising complete natural movements and maintaining a good posture through all your activities, you should not require much stretching to maintain good muscle length. Certainly, I don't think Maerk spent much time stretching, but then he never let his level of flexibility get as poor as most people have…

Warm up

With that point in mind, **warming up** before workouts is probably a good idea, but there is an embarrassing deficit of evidence to back-up the claim that stretching reduces the likelihood of injury. If you are going to stretch before workouts, you need to know that exercise science has moved on from the days when static stretches were recommended. It is almost universally accepted now that *dynamic exercises* are preferable. You wouldn't guess this if you watch the warm-up at many grass-level sports clubs where you still see players trying to balance on one foot, pulling the other up behind their thigh in an attempt to give it a good pre-workout stretch. This has been shown to tire the muscles unnecessarily and reduce coordination and performance.

If there is still any case to be made for this sort of static, yoga-like exercise, then it is post-workout or between workouts; never before.

The best way to warm up is to go through the same movements that you will be making in the main phase of the warm-up, albeit more slowly, with less weight and with fewer repetitions. This will prepare the mind, warm the muscles, increase the range of movement and raise the pulse for the exertion that is to follow.

Going Hardcore

If you have completely bought into my analysis of Maerk's day and the need to have an exercise schedule (and indeed a lifestyle) that resembles it, then you may be wondering if there isn't value in constructing a workout that resembles even more closely the challenges that hunter-gatherers faced. Would it not be better to actually train in the forest using logs, fallen trees, rocks, branches, streams, and the natural environment as our training equipment?

The answer is an unequivocal and resounding 'Yes!' It's an amazing experience and, mixed with a spirit of playfulness and exploration, can change the way you think about exercise and fitness forever. For those for whom the call of the forest beckons, there is a whole new level of contact with our human roots to be gained from training in this way.

This form of training (or more accurately, self-development) is growing increasingly popular and it's almost single-handedly down to the efforts of an inspiring Frenchman called **Erwan Le Corre**. His video on YouTube, 'The Workout that Time Forgot', might be *the* most inspirational training montage ever filmed! (See **www.movnat.com**)

MovNat training brings people together to run, jump, climb, balance, jump, swim, lift, carry, and even fight. They concentrate on these natural movements in all of their training and it's considered by its adherents to be the most functional form of training available.

I have taken many clients into the forest to train and they love it. We've lifted logs, carried rocks, climbed boulders, crawled up slopes, pulled ourselves up and onto branches, jumped streams – and had some sensational sessions.

Is this essential? No. Is it preferable? Maybe. The movement patterns may be more random and diverse, which has to be good; but it's an individual thing. We don't all have to get right back to nature in all its mucky glory to get the most of the benefits available to us. Also, many people have lost the ability to express themselves spontaneously in this way. It would need a whole other book to put most people on track with this way of being, thinking and moving.

I love what Erwan Le Corre does and I love why he does it. When we met, I told him this. Many of the points I've expressed come out of principles we both share. In fact, I would like to train the way he does more often, but it takes a greater leap of faith for many clients to adopt this approach in the conservative setting of the Home Counties. However, for practicality's sake and to keep this book realistic for the typical reader, I stopped short of these more radical recommendations.

In writing this book, I wanted to write a resource for everyone, so I have stopped shy of recommending that people dispense with formal training entirely and spend their time playfully pursuing natural movements in natural environments. If you do – please give me a call and tell me where you're playing and I might just come and join you!

I hope that the routines I outline in the book represent something that people can start doing today, right now... and that was always my aim when I started this project.

Chapter Key points

- *Movement is life: looking to improve the quantity and quality of our movement has to be a central axiom of any approach to a better and longer life.*

- *Our bodies expect natural movement (not gym movement), so make your movements as much like Maerk's as possible.*

- *Concentrate on cardio strength, aerobic capacity and posture flexibility; add additional elements like pure strength, speed, balance, agility when and if necessary.*

- *Build movement into your day or start a regular circuit routine.*

- *Skip any extended cardio work (running, rowing etc) that leaves you breathing heavily for more than 15 minutes.*

- *Instead perform high-intensity 'Emergency Training' up to two times a week. Sprint training is ideal.*

- *Include 3-5 hours of low-key aerobic movement into your week. Walking is fine, or any low-stress sport.*

- *Combine your exercise (especially sprints) with a missed meal for amazing fat-burning results.*

References:

La Gerche A, et al "Exercise-induced right ventricular dysfunction and structural remodelling in endurance athletes" Europena Heart Journal 2011; DOI: 10.1093/eurheartj/ehr397.

Tabata I, Nishimura K, Kouzaki M, et al. (1996) "Effects of moderate-intensity endurance and high-intensity intermittent training on anaerobic capacity and VO$_2$max". Med Sci Sports Exerc 28(10): 1327–30.

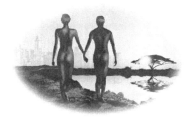

CHAPTER NINE

Natural Posture

*"If one's posture is upright, one has no
need to fear a crooked shadow"*

Unknown

The Collapse of Modern Society.

The movements and eating patterns described in the previous chapters are all essential elements, but for maximum performance and comfortable longevity, there's something else we must consider. Maerk, you see, had the advantage of a posture free from the deformities caused by modern comforts, his body still working just how evolution intended.

I know good posture is not something that gets talked about much anymore, and you may now be thinking I'm going in a stiff and starchy direction here, but you'll soon find out that posture is the essential foundation on which our IF pyramid is built.

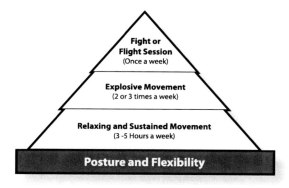

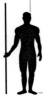

Imagine one of those great big tower cranes you see looming over a city skyline. Imagine its girder framework standing straight and strong, lifting heavy loads effortlessly and in great safety. Now imagine you're standing at the bottom watching it at work when you notice its girder framework is badly twisted and bent. There's a great bow in its central pillar warping the whole structure. Someone has even offset the cab right at the top in a vain attempt to keep it balanced. You're shocked to hear it creak and groan alarmingly when it lifts a heavy load. How safe do you feel standing there?

Fancy a trip up to the cab?

Spinal Collapse

Most individuals suffer – knowingly or not – from a collapse in their spinal structure. In most people, the spine, which is the foundation of our life-long fight against gravity, is in nowhere near the state it evolved to be. In the western, developed world there are very few exceptions to this. Spinal collapse is one of the most debilitating conditions affecting our society today and this leads to a number of issues:

- *Pain (in the back or 'referred pain' to the knees, hips and other areas)*
- *Reduced health (our internal organs become damaged through compression)*
- *Fatigue and reduced zest for life*
- *Reduced mobility, muscle imbalances and flexibility problems*
- *Lack of co-ordination, efficiency and reduced sporting performance (It's no coincidence that the best athletes are those who frequently exhibit the very best spinal health and postures: look at Kenyan distance runners or Jamaican sprinters.)*
- *An unattractive look*

Before we look at what can be done about this, let's see if we can pin down what we're talking about. The most obvious way you will know that your spine is out of kilter is that your back hurts – it really is that simple. We've come to accept back pain as a normal fact of life, but it shouldn't be. If it does hurt, even periodically, you're not alone and you are sharing the experience of the 95% of the developed world.

> It is interesting to note that even without medical care, drugs and therapists, large swathes of the developing world have less than 5% occurrences of back pain, even when engaged in a lifetime of heavy labour. There are ladies in Africa and Asia who spend up to 10 hours a week working bent over in paddy fields who report no difficulties with maintaining this position and continue to work in this way into old age. A typical westerner could not work for more than a couple of hours before their bent spine would be racked with pain...

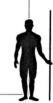

If you have back pain – usually lower-back pain – you experience first-hand the effects of this almost universal western malaise. Others might only rarely suffer back pain and not notice its insidious effects. Even if you feel like you're in good health, you will find (assuming your posture is less than good) that there are clues that you are in less than good alignment.

Try thinking about the following:

1. *Do you find standing for longer periods of time tiring?*

2. *Do you find yourself slumping lower in your chair as time passes?*

3. *Do you find that you store tension in your shoulders? Maybe you have a tension 'knot' between your neck and your shoulders?*

4. *Do you find yourself off balance when you reach for things?*

5. *Do your knees hurt or click when they bend? Do your heels come off the floor when you squat onto your haunches?*

6. *Do you feel your head tries to disappear into your neck when you bend over? Can you keep your back straight when bending forward from the hips (like the ladies who work in the fields I mentioned earlier)? Or does your upper body curl over like a large letter 'C'?*

7. *Hold your arms extended above your head in front of a mirror. Now squat until your knees are parallel. Notice:*

   a) Do your knees move out smoothly over the second toes of each foot as they should, or do they pitch inwards (knock-kneed)?

b) Do your arms stay vertically above your head, or are you forced to lower them as you squat?

c) If you can keep your arms vertical, can you still squat fully and comfortably without arching your mid-back?

8. Do you have difficulties turning your head fully (90 degrees) to the left or right without also moving either shoulder?

Testing by Appearances

With practice you can look at someone and see if they hold themselves in good alignment. We can think of the different segments of our body as building blocks. Like any sort of structure (imagine a stack of cardboard boxes in a warehouse), it only has integrity when each block is balanced properly over the others. If one segment is out of kilter, all the rest must be too in order to maintain any sort of balance. Like building bricks, any deviance from the perfect stack results in instability and structural weakness. In the case of our bodies, we require additional energy and tension in the muscles to remain upright. It also results in an unpleasing asymmetry.

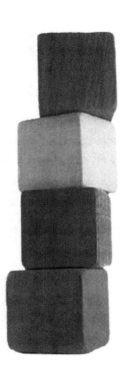

How to check your posture

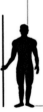

Take a photo of yourself in profile (use a mirror if necessary) wearing only your underclothes. Open it up in a programme like Photoshop, or just print it so you can draw on it. Now draw a plumb line straight upward (90° perpendicular to the floor, parallel with any walls) from your heels, straight through whatever is vertically above it.

If you are in good alignment, the line should pass through the ankle, knee, hip bone, shoulder and ear like it does on the figure on the left, below.

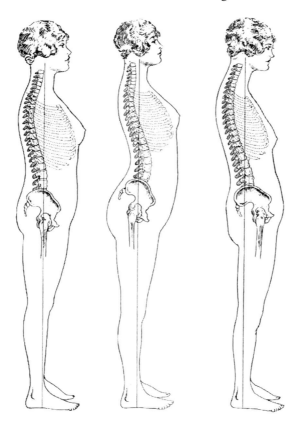

If it does, congratulations - you are one of the few people I know who is able to stand (and most likely move too) in good alignment with good posture and poise. Most people in the UK, Europe and North America (i.e. most of those living in the developed world) *will* fail this test.

What is correct posture?

Many people who are concerned or proud of their posture make an effort to correct it. Typically, they find themselves standing or sitting slumped over and then resolve to brace themselves 'upright'. Many people have been making this 'correction' movement for so long they are no longer aware that they spend all day hauling themselves upright.

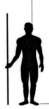

> The military teaches its recruits to force themselves into 'good posture' from day one. Unfortunately these efforts are all based around a false premise: that additional effort can overcome the underlying problem of malcoordination.

There is no one, fixed position for the human body to assume, but there will always be some recognisably 'right' positions under certain fixed conditions.

One such condition is standing still. If you can do this well, without fixing yourself into that position, you will instantly and instinctively make the minimum adjustments needed to cope with additional challenges, such as bending, jumping or walking.

As the old adage says, we must 'learn to walk before we run'; in the same way we must learn to stand before we can walk – there is a natural hierarchy to these things. Learning to stand well, sit well, and even lie well is essential if your body is to retain or regain the natural symmetry that will keep you pain free, healthy, efficient and relaxed.

Maybe you think you have these qualities already? Maybe people have told you that you have 'great posture' or you just don't ever get back pain, hip pain, shoulder ache – or any of these things I've listed?

So how is your posture?

Take another look at your whole-body profile shot in Photoshop (the one with your plumb line).

Look for these things:

Do any of the key markers I listed above fall out of line with that plumb line? If they do – even just one of them – there are things you need to work on. Even if you think all those markers line up down the plumb-line, it's possible that you are using far too much effort to hold yourself in a fixed, immobile position.

The most likely thing you will see is that your hips are pushed well forward of the marker line. If that's the case, it's almost certain that your head will be too. You will experience **Forward Head Syndrome** in almost every movement.

Here is a young teenager whose spine is already clearly bent out of shape by gravity:

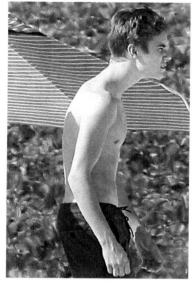

Forward Head Syndrome

It's actually American boy-singer and teenage heart-throb, Justin Bieber. (You may not have heard of him if you're not female and younger than about 14 - but if this posture becomes habitual, he won't keep his millions of screaming fans for long!) If you remember Arun copying his father's movements, what kind of example is this icon of teenage vitality unintentionally setting for our youth? Though, to be honest, all the best people have had this problem, as I used to carry my head a bit like this too.

Having pointed this out, you will probably try to fix the problem by holding your head in a different manner. Don't. You will just add another layer of tension over the layers you already carry. Your head (your uppermost balance block) is misplaced because the blocks underneath it are misplaced too. Your head needs to go where it is at present because, without adding yet more tension, you will just fall over if it goes elsewhere - and that would look even sillier!

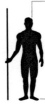

Your head is probably leaning forward to counterbalance
your back… which is too far behind the plumb line…
because your pelvis is too far in front of the plumb line…
because … oh, you get the idea.

Consider now why this sort of intervention is necessary. Why are so many of us bent out of shape like this? Why are so many of us being sentenced to an old age where we can only shuffle along looking at the ground?

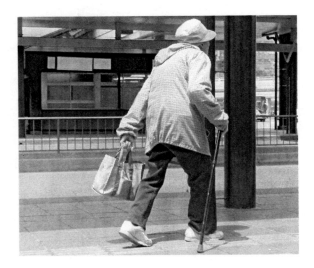

We have already looked at one obvious reason for this malady: a sedentary existence. The term has two meanings, both of which are applicable. We often use the term to denote a life without much movement. This is certainly a contributing factor in this epidemic of badly-stacked people. So in effect, lack of movement leads to inflexibility and weakness, whereas flexibility and strength are required to align well. Got it?

Get off your backside!

The other sense in which we are sedentary is the more literal interpretation: we sit, sit, sit, and sit. Here it's not just the inherent lack of movement that is a problem while we are sitting; it's the actual process of sitting itself that's so harmful to us.

Sitting is a modern aberration. In fact, most people in the world don't sit and don't want to. I'm sure you know that if you visit Africa or Asia, you will find most people opt automatically and naturally for an alternative resting position: **the squat.**

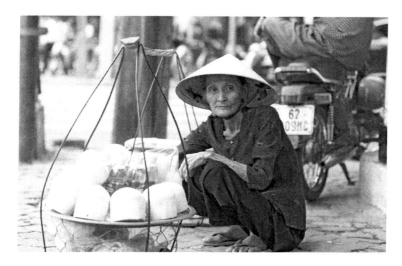

To people from countries that haven't yet fallen for the charms of the armchair and who are well practiced in squatting from childhood through their whole lives, squatting isn't hard at all. They find it easy and restful – a position they can sit in for hours.

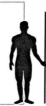

And it's not actually just the less developed nations that consider sitting on chairs to be an anathema. Consider the Japanese, an affluent, sophisticated country. They continue to prefer to kneel at low tables rather than to place their (usually well-aligned) spines on chairs. Like the traditions in Africa and Asia, this position is part of their ancient culture, in which traditional resting positions have remained unchanged for thousands of years.

In the western world – yet again – things are different. As soon as chairs became available, they were seized upon as a form of status symbol. To be raised off the ground (on a throne, to take the ultimate symbol of power) was to be exalted over those that sat beneath you.

The issue with chairs is that they need a high level of physical awareness to be used properly without slow, almost unnoticeable, damage to your posture, spine and balance. Over time, the poor use of chairs reduces your ability not only to sit properly, but to stand properly, walk properly, and even to lie down beneficially to rest.

> Babies and very young children can sit in a reasonably well designed chair pretty well. And so can about 1 in 300 adults. But most people can't – and they suffer badly for that fact.

Interestingly, this hasn't always been the case. You might expect me to tell you that the rot set in from the very first moment a human sat on a chair, but you'd be wrong.

It seems that chairs have only been as harmful as they are for about 70 to 90 years. In order for the full harmful effects of hours a day in a chair to be felt, something else is needed too: diminished kinaesthetic awareness (our sense of what it feels like to be in good alignment).

When this becomes impaired (through factors we'll look at soon) the presence of chairs in our lives seriously exacerbates any issues in a vicious circle that lowers our physical capacity considerably. We have issues – so we sit badly – so the issues worsen – so we sit worse... And so the cycle continues.

As I've suggested, our diminished kinaesthetic awareness dates back not to the advent of agriculture, as you might expect me to say, but only for less than a century. I suspect that the alignment of hunter-gatherers was better than most of those who worked in fields; however, the biggest change occurred only in the 1920s.

As many of you will know, until recently a part of every young lady's education was deportment lessons. This acknowledges the importance given by society at this time to the quality of standing well and moving well. We talked about people moving with 'grace and poise' – terms that are generally out of favour today. Perhaps they sound a bit old-fashioned or elitist to us?

Not all of the training given to young people and the practice they sustained in later life was of a first class nature, but the point is that there used to be an awareness of what it meant to be well-aligned. In the upper classes this awareness was consciously recognised and strived for; in other classes it was perhaps less of a conscious consideration, but still very much a feature of everyday living.

Like Arun, we cannot help but want to copy those around us. If they stand well, sit well, and move with grace and poise, then so will we. Our elders set the example and we follow. We are easily conditioned creatures until we make a conscious effort to change ourselves.

The 1930s had a depression – but the 20s had their own slump!

Around 1920, a greater influence than the good example of our parents and grandparents hit the scene: the media. The mass production of magazines and newspapers meant that new influences had a chance to infiltrate our lives. In this case, the expanding influence of the fashion industry and the power of publishing created a new sense of identity for upwardly mobile adults.

Suddenly, new images were flashed around the world - enticing pictures of 'cool', snazzy, debonair young men and women. They were startling in appearance: they looked different, acted differently, spoke differently, danced differently, and dressed differently; however they also *stood* differently, *sat* differently and *walked* differently. All these things marked them out as 'bright young things' and 'young thrusters' – and they became the poster boys and girls of a new generation.

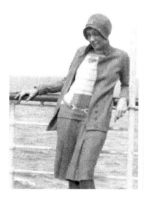 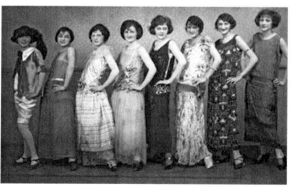

If you have ever looked at old black and white photographs (pre-1920) you might have been struck by how rigid and stiff characters in portraits and group photos look compared with those we might see today. You might think how uptight, fixed and straight this pre-Great War generation looks to our modern sensibilities. You might take this as evidence of how much more 'relaxed' we are these days. You might also conclude that there is a connection between our more open, less hierarchical society and the stiff, inflexible way this older generation appear to hold themselves. Their lives look more sombre and serious than ours.

Certainly I had all these thoughts for years, but I now believe this is an absolute fallacy. If there is such a thing as odd behaviour, it is our modern manner.

There's no doubt that this 'black and white' generation had to take life seriously, but surely we do too? In terms of the 'unnatural' rigidity we see in the photos, we simply misunderstand how the nature of photograph taking has changed over the years. In fact I would say it is *us* who are the anomaly; it is us who have become incredibly casual in front of the lens and put ourselves into positions that, though normal to us, are historically and anatomically odd.

Nowadays we take photos casually at the drop of a hat, often with mobile phones. For the Victorians and Edwardians, having a portrait photo taken was an expensive, lengthy and formal affair. If one was lucky enough to appear in a photo it was deemed very important to take the opportunity to appear as dignified as possible; dignity demands *formality*, and formality dictates that one should adopt one's very best pose. Naturally these individuals adopted the poses that they had been taught from an early age were the 'right' ones for persons of 'good standing' (pun intended). A good model was there to follow and, naturally, when the marvel of the camera appeared only the very best pose would do.

Away from the camera they wouldn't have been as strict with themselves, but the baseline positions of good posture that we observe in these photos would have been ever present in their lives.

The fact that these individuals maintained good posture throughout their lives is evident in the photos and portraits we have as records. Even though bank clerks (to take an example) might have been required to sit down for up to 12 hours a day, they were capable of doing so without any form of spinal collapse and without the sort of degeneration and pain that is so prevalent today.

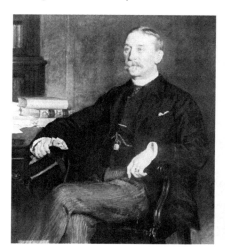 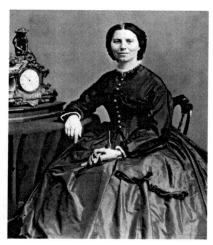

This almost lost generation knew how to sit properly, how to stand properly, how to walk properly – and not even the harmful habit of continual sitting was enough to throw them wildly off-kilter.

However, the cultural shift of the 1920s was to change all of that. A brave new generation threw out the old adages, images and examples of their forbearers and set out into the world with a new, daring demeanour: the slouch.

I want to look now at what they actually started to do with their anatomy. In doing so we will start to see what we can do to rectify matters in our own lives. Their problems are *our* problems, you see. It will become apparent why an intention (or admonition) to 'sit up straight' is really of no help to us.

A very modern stance

You'll come to see that many of the positions we think looked relaxed and comfortable are actually nothing of the sort. They are dominated by a level of tension and discomfort that we have learnt to ignore and accept as normal. **Again, we have lost our instincts.**

Unfortunately, in a book of this sort, it isn't possible to do much more than outline the changes that you could make over a few weeks that would radically transform your relation to gravity. In brief though, there are a series of closely-related habits that almost all of us have. These are:

1. *We push our pelvis forward.*

2. *We rock forward so our weight goes over our toes, rather than our heels.*

3. *Our shoulders fall forward, downwards and towards each other (the 'slump') to compensate for our forward-positioned pelvis. (Hump-backed celebrity Quasimodo models this well, but he has many lesser imitators!)*

4. *Our head juts forward to compensate for the backward-positioned shoulders.*

The technical name for this is 'kyphosis'. Here is a particularly bad case:

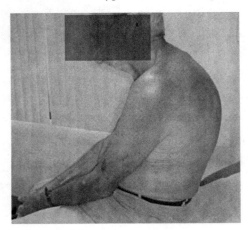

On top of this, the following often happens:

1. *The arches of the foot roll in (There is some suggestion that this excessive movement – known as hyper-pronation - could be a congenital issue, but there's plenty of evidence that poor posture and poor shoes are also to blame. We will talk more about shoes later.)*

2. *Because of this your knees fall towards each other when you bend them instead of tracking straight over the toes (you become 'knock-kneed').*

3. *Lots of muscles and joints stiffen up (too many to list here).*

4. *Some muscles and joints become hyper-flexible to compensate for the joints that barely move at all.*

5. *Your walking gait becomes odd: you lean forwards or backwards unnecessarily; you stiffen your legs unnecessarily and you throw your feet out in front of you. You may lurch from side-to-side or bounce up-and-down as you walk. (Check by walking towards a mirror – your head should glide forward as if on rails)*

People are often aware that something is amiss – consciously or not – and many do the following to try to negate the issues described above:

1. *You pull your head back again (to stand 'straight') and your chin IN.*

2. *You puff out your chest and heave your torso up and backwards (to avoid the slouch).*

3. *You suck your stomach in (you think it makes you look thinner too).*

4. *You lock your knees out.*

I call the second adaption 'military posture'. If you were in the military you almost certainly do this (unless you ignored your drill sergeant's instructions) but so do lots of people who make a deliberate effort to stand-up straight.

These last two adaptions lead to one or more of the following:

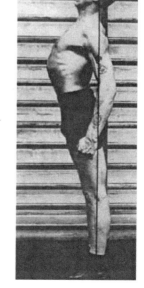

1. *A hollow lower back (known as lordosis)*

2. *A bum that disappears inside your trousers, so that your trousers just hang off the back of your belt.*

3. *Lots of additional tension – mental and physical – which is even more than the amount required to hold the slouch position (hence the dichotomy between the terms 'ATTENTION' and 'AT EASE' in military parlance. These should be the same thing when an individual is well balanced.)*

Military stance: many people's idea of how to stand straighter. Notice however, that the hips and chest are much too far in front of the plumb line.

People who have grabbed the bull by the horns and pulled themselves by the bootstraps into what they believe is a better position often look like their posture is better than those who don't; they may even receive regular compliments from acquaintances. However, those compliments are just noting the absence of the *appearance* of the sort of slouch we are used to seeing, and it assumes that what has replaced it is optimal or preferable. In truth, either situation is harmful - however much the 'military posture' might look more pleasing to some eyes.

Here are some pictures of relatively modern but traditional people standing or moving well. Each body segment is stacked up perfectly over the next, the shoulders are well back and aligned, and their poise radiates grace and confidence.

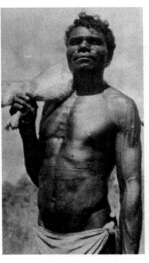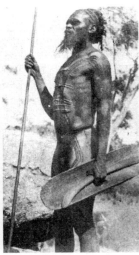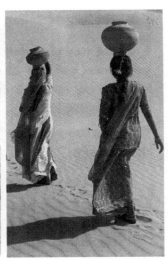

You'll see from this that most of those who have grown up without western sedentary patterns of movement are much more likely to retain good body alignment – even into old age.

I would surmise that this is for the following reasons.

1. *They are active for much of the day.*

2. *They don't slouch about on chairs.*

3. *They go barefoot much of the time over varying terrain and retain strength and flexibility in their feet. They certainly don't totter about in high-heels or cushioned trainers, which encourages a horrible displacement of the pelvis!*

4. *They squat regularly and retain flexibility even as they age.*

5. *They don't sleep on soft mattresses, which smothers the body's ability to sense where it is in space and relax properly. It also encourages the body to curl up in a 'C'-shaped, foetus position (a position surprisingly suitable only for foetuses!)*

6. *They retain strength across all muscle groupings, not just those isolated at the gym.*

7. *They are rarely obese. (Obesity makes it even harder to fight against gravity once you are at all off-balance).*

8. *They have inherited an ancient culture of good posture which each new generation learns from the last.*

Based on this, I would make the following general suggestions with regard to posture, flexibility and the good movement patterns that stem from this:

1. *Become more aware of your current posture and tension levels. By doing so you will be able to consciously let go of some of the excess effort you are using.*

2. *Learn how to sit well in a chair so you can sit on most chairs for hours without issue when you have to. Learn how to stand well. Learn how to lie in your bed while decompressing your spinal joints and resting fully.*

3. *Squat more often. Before you can squat properly with your heels flat on the ground, you may have to work up to it by squatting with your heels raised on a block.*

4. *Stand or walk around at work when you can. (In California, lots of office workers have begun standing at their workstations rather than sitting!)*

5. *Go barefoot when you can: on holiday; on the beach; around the house. Buy shoes with plenty of lateral toe space, no heels and a thin sole. (I train, work and live in a special pair of shoes called Vibram FiveFingers. They're amazing, but you'd be a brave man to wear them to the office!)*

6. *Consider a new mattress – not too hard, not too soft. ('Too hard' just means you can't get used to it and sleep eludes you… and you should have gathered by now that you do need your sleep!)*

7. *Regain lost flexibility – to help you lose these patterns of excess tension and tightness the years have brought you could consider massage, a specific dynamic stretching routine prescribed just for you by a human movement expert, using a foam roller, or even inversion therapy. (However, once you've learnt how to integrate these superior habits of poise into your life you probably won't need these modern aids)*

8. *Learn what good posture looks like, practice to achieve it, and then teach your children!*

Posture might not be 'cool' or in any way 'rock n roll' but to hold what is an evolutionary correct body position does bring numerous benefits to our lives.

Great posture also promotes great flexibility, and together they create a noticeably superior level of structural integrity and strength. Like it or not, 'posture' is undoubtedly the unshakable base upon which all physical movements are built. Most of the best athletes the world has known have had postures that set them apart from the common riff-raff.

So hang your jeans low and adopt a fashionable 'street' slump for a night on the tiles by all means; but, come morning, please re-adopt the stance nature intended!

The next chapter will pull the rug out from under the feet of the fitness industry's answer to everything: that paying for a gym subscription is the one-stop shop for health and wellbeing.

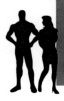

Chapter Key points

- *Relearn good posture to remain mobile for an extra decade or two*
- *Squat more often*
- *Avoid chairs where possible until you can sit properly*
- *Find opportunities to exercise barefooted or in minimalist shoes*

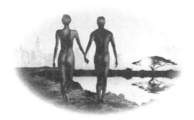

CHAPTER TEN

The Gym Won't Help (Much)

"Whoso would be a man,
must be a non-conformist"

Ralph Waldo Emerson

The florescent lit, pounding music, lycra-donning fiesta that is the local gym is often considered by many people to be the number one resource to improve themselves physically. With many thousands of people handing over their credit card details for a subscription each year, a modern gym jammed full of fancy-looking machinery that goes 'beep' and a slick sales team to make grand promises is all too often seen as the easiest route to our modern day quest for fitness. In fact, I consider it the biggest sidetrack many people will take on their path to a fully functioning body.

One of the biggest problems with gyms is that, with all those machines churning away in such a predicable repetitious manner, they're actually just not that much fun. So after the initial enthusiasm-filled visits the shine quickly wears off, the excuses *not* to go are soon being pulled out of the bag more often than the sweat bands.

It is part and parcel of the business model of the gym that enrols you that you're going to quickly stop going – but to avoid the stigma of being shown up as a proven quitter, you're unlikely to be brave enough to cancel your subscription.

The reasons people quit are many, but most boil down to two simple points:

1. *They don't like going.*
2. *They don't achieve the results they want.*

If that sounds like you, then the first thing you need to know is that it's not your fault. I bet that comes as quite a relief, doesn't it? As I will show you as you read on, the cards are inordinately stacked against you when it comes to following this conveniently packaged path to fitness.

Seriously, it's not your fault if you're fat, and it's not your fault if you don't like the gym, don't exercise, don't like your body, or can't get the results you want – and I'll tell you why.

There's little in a gym that connects with a human being's innate instincts, other than their unfortunate propensity to be attracted towards the empty promise of a quick fix. That's why it's both so hard to get results and so hard to keep going.

Ultimately, you should accept that commercial gyms are founded on a business model that doesn't try as hard to help you as it does to separate you from your cash. However, to be fair, the modern gym wasn't actually developed with you in mind at all.

In pursuit of... 'muscliness'

Long before 'normal' people went to gyms, machines like the ones you see in every modern gym facility were developed for making muscles all big and puffy – for obtaining that certain macho appearance. People who liked this look and adopted this hobby became known as 'bodybuilders'. They are a very specific type of person with very specific needs: usually men looking for a very particular 'extreme;' look. Body building isn't about health; it isn't about flexibility or stamina, energy or even strength. It's just about huge muscles.

Body builders don't want to feel healthier. They don't want to move better. They don't even want to be any stronger. There's nothing in particular they want to be able to do better except to look better in a posing pouch.

There is nothing that they won't do in the pursuit of greater muscle mass. They will take dangerous steroids that compromise their health; eat huge quantities of food of dubious quality; and often refrain from any other form of exercise at all lest they burn precious calories they need for muscle growth. They will spend money on fake tan and baby oil, which they will cover themselves with – anything that will get them closer to their ideal muscle-bound image.

To achieve this look, special machines were developed that were capable of isolating each muscle. Over the last 30 years, however, these same machines have been used to commercialise the gym 'experience', convincing a wider public that these facilities fulfil our need for regular movement. Despite throwing the doors open to a wider public, gyms remain a facility designed for the likes of these bodybuilding men, not for meeting the needs of more typical individuals who desire weight loss, strength, balance, flexibility and better health.

So really, it's horses for courses. If you're looking for humungous muscles, get down the gym, get on the 'pec-deck' or Smith machine, and make sure you take whatever sugar-filled meal-replacement packet they want to sell you too! If however you want to be agile, supple, energetic, stronger, leaner and fitter in a real world way, perhaps you need to look elsewhere.

The blind leading the blind

Go into almost any gym in the country and you'll see the same thing: people dabbling about nervously; people fighting strong feelings of self-consciousness (reinforced by ubiquitous mirrors); people doubting what they are doing and wondering what on earth they are doing there. As a gym newbie, we suspect everyone else knows what they are doing and is quietly laughing at us.

With a bit more time spent learning the ropes, we inevitably settle in and those feelings subside, often to be replaced with those of boredom. We wrongly thought in the early days that we would grow to like it when we saw results, but sooner rather than later the realisation dawns that our dream of a miraculous body transformation isn't just around the corner.

Typically we'll have been diligently following the routine set up by a gym instructor. Probably one with only a few weeks training who, even if he knows better, has little option but to prescribe the exercises he has been told he should include in everyone's programme. He might tell you that his programme is just for you, but actually, like a cog in the machine, he churns out the same exercises for *every* gym member, merely varying the number of reps and sets depending on whether you described yourself as a beginner or an intermediate in your induction.

Most of the exercises he'll get you to do will be one of two types a) largely useless, or b) dangerous. Most exercises will be of type 'a' – a few are type 'b'. The only exception to the uselessness of the programme is if you are actually a bodybuilder and are beginning a serious, six-meal-a-day, extreme nutritional programme to try and inflate your muscles to look a bit stronger. What a waste of time *and* money!

So there you are, blindly following a gym routine founded on repetition, routine, drudgery, ineffectiveness and a little old-fashioned narcissism because you know no better.

So you might wonder why it's come to this. Well it's quite simple. From the gym owners' point of view this system works *brilliantly*. They carefully set up a system to charge people to stay away from their gym and not use their facilities. This is exactly what most gym members do; they stay at home. They don't use the gym because they don't actually like it and, deep down in their gut work, they know it won't work for them.

However, they don't cancel their membership because to do so would be to admit defeat – to concede that they will never get fit again and that they've failed. So they carry on paying for a service that they don't use in the vain hope that one day they'll return. Statistically 80% of gym users are absent on any given day from the gym for which they pay an on-going membership.

This suits the gym owner just fine. In fact, their worst nightmare is that gym becomes popular and everyone starts turning up. They haven't possibly got room. Instead, they hope that the *idea* of the gym stays popular; that the belief that the gym is the only way to a better quality of wellbeing stays entrenched in our conditioned minds so they can continue to charge us for this state of affairs. But *should* you have the gall to turn up, they then want to squeeze a bit more out of your pocket by selling you some *more* stuff that you really don't need: dodgy protein shakes, snack bars, supplements, and the services of 'personal trainers' who will follow you around watching you do the same exercises you've always done.

Strength is an all-in team effort

The obvious thing that anybody with eyes in their head will quickly notice is that gyms are filled with machines. The machines purport to get you fit, one muscle at a time. Each is designed to isolate individual muscles and exercise them separately from the surrounding ones.

Isn't it ironic that people go to the gym to get mobile again? All the machines are static and fixed to the floor. There's little genuine movement to be seen at all!

Take, for example, the leg extension machine. This is a bench over which your leg hangs. The leg is then extended until it is straight whilst overcoming the inertia posed by the weight resisting this movement. It mainly works one muscle: the Rectus Femoris. Yet at the front of your upper leg alone there are 6 different muscles, and each must work together in unison to be effective in any real-life task or sport. So in fact the exact circumstances that this machine contrives to produce – where one muscle stands alone to do all the work – don't exist anywhere else.

Typically, the result of this sort of training is that the targeted muscle becomes filled with additional fluids, making it look bigger and stronger – though increases in actual strength are often minimal. When this happens, you are, for a brief moment, a bodybuilder.

Now this might not sound too bad a compromise for the ease of using a nice machine. But here's the thing. This sort of exercise is totally unnatural. There is nothing else you will *ever* do in your life where your leg operates in this way. Think back to Maerk's daily life. He doesn't do anything like this. All of his movements involve moving or carrying an object along an unprescribed, non-linear route. To do this he had to coordinate all the muscles of his body at the same time, balancing himself whilst creating the force necessary to make his intended movement, and he did so with grace, efficiency and great posture.

In any real life movement our body works as a whole. Almost all of the other muscles contribute to assist balance and support the whole body for every movement we make. Machines, however, isolate muscles and fix our joints in space apart from the one being worked. In doing so, they produce a response which does not improve anything other than the quality of 'puffiness' that the targeted muscle exhibits, and a marginally-elevated ability to perform *just that one exercise.*

> Think of muscle isolation exercises as being like training a regiment of soldiers at home on a distance learning package, and expecting them to march in time on pass out day!

If you've ever wondered how after a 12-week gym programme you still find it just as hard to lift the shopping out of the boot, here's your answer: you've hardly improved the strength of any whole groups of muscles at all – and there's been no improvement in the *synchronisation* of the muscle groups involved in this whole body lifting task. Strength is just as much about improved co-ordination as it is about genuine muscle growth. The swollen muscle effect may look very impressive, but it's little more than that. Essentially it's a vanity project.

In this sort of environment no learning happens and there's no real engagement with the environment. Our gym user knows the machine will work exactly as it did last time and that there is no need to be fully present in mind and body in the same way that Maerk is when he engages fully with a task while keeping his awareness open for threats at all times.

So, why are gyms filled with machines if they aren't much use to most of us? It's simple really; the reason is that this is the only way that they can justify the prices they charge. They give you something very obvious to see when you enter the gym and, if you believe that using such machines is the only useful way to exercise, it reinforces the idea that you can't possibly get fit on your own. After all, where would you put all the machines that are needed?

Gyms are good for cardio right?

Ah, but what about the **'cardio' machines**, I hear you ask. Surely the stair climber, the cross trainer, and the stationery cycle are good for burning off fat and strengthening my heart and lungs? Well, maybe. I would be mad to suggest that you'd be better off at home on the sofa, but I still have some serious reservations about these machines.

Firstly, they're dull. Duller than a dull day in Dulwich! Being stationery, you are faced with an unchanging view for long periods of time. This really isn't very natural. You've probably noticed that when you walk or cycle outdoors normally, the scenery tends to trundle on past you? Not so in the gym. You do sometimes get given a mini-television to watch though. This will ensure that there is no way that your mind can be fully involved in the present moment and engaged with the activity you are mindlessly pursuing.

Secondly, you're indoors, yet cardiovascular exercise presents the best opportunity to get outside the concrete cages we surround ourselves with all day long. Getting outdoors, ideally into a natural environment, is one of the most crucial things to do to boost your metabolic rate and raise serotonin and Vitamin D levels. This is hardly an arcane secret: it's not only backed by science but also the good instincts of those city office workers who try to get to the park in their lunch break. They know from experience that their afternoon will be the better for it with higher levels of energy, motivation and drive.

What is less well known is that there is a growing number of people attesting to the existence of "Nature Deficit Disorder" which appears to affect many people who don't get a sufficient dose of mud, leaves, trees, insects, wind, temperature change, sunshine and other facets of a real environment – all the things that Maerk interacted with every day of his life.

Others have dismissed the idea that this should be considered a disorder, citing a lack of evidence. All I know is that most of the happy times of my life have been outdoors, and I think that's no coincidence. I am always happier at the end of a walk in the woods than I am when I set off. Never have I returned to the house miserable, wishing I'd covered the same distance inside at a gym.

Thirdly, most of these machines, apart from the treadmill, are *non-weight bearing*. Now this can be a good thing if you are injured. However it's well known that an absence of weight-bearing activity leads to a weakening of the bones and connective tissues, and increased incidences of falls and broken bones in later life. So it is just possible that the cross-trainer isn't the wonder machine it is often painted as.

My fourth reason is that the machines are so often used competitively. We compete with ourselves and we compete with the person next to us. This isn't useful for cardio. Cardio should be conducted at an easy, conversational pace so that we finish feeling more energised than when we started. However, gyms and the nature of cardio machines encourage us to push, push and push – until we're ready to drop.

Now this isn't something a human being should choose to do regularly. If you're not sure about this, check out the health record of most world-class endurance athletes. Despite being awesomely fit, they are often on the edge of breakdown, with their immune systems stretched to the limit to counter the physical and mental stresses to which they subject themselves. Maerk would not have seen the point of this and would have sensibly chosen to save his energy for emergencies or activities with more intrinsic meaning.

Finally, all cardio is mechanistic. Even on the treadmill – yes, you're running which is good – but every step is exactly like the last. The ground underneath your feet is identical for every pace meaning the tiny muscles in your feet are not encouraged to work hard to adjust to constantly changing terrain, as Maerk's are when he crosses stony, uneven ground. Your balance is never challenged.

Beware of your metabolism

Now I'm certainly not against running. I love it. What I see as harmful is the 'chronic' form of cardio (in the form of running, bicycling, or whatever) that most people adopt. If you're out of breath for extended periods of time, you're doing yourself no long-term favours. You can't even expect to burn off more fat this way. At higher speeds our metabolism switches from burning fat as its primary fuel, to glucose.

This means that glucose (the sugar that gets stored in the muscles) gets depleted, a situation that our body doesn't take kindly to. Its response is to desperately recoup what's been lost and to do its best to prevent this situation happening again. So it increases appetite over the next 24 hours.

The result of all this stock depletion is: **You end up actually eating *more* after this sort of exercise and often add MORE weight to your poor frame.** I have read that the average body fat percentage of runners at running clubs is 22% (a bit chubby). Should we not expect this to be much lower if regular, extended, effortful running was a helpful adjunct to weight loss?

Therefore, as a rule of thumb, when exercise is extensive (25 minutes plus) it should be so dead easy that, should you choose, you could keep at it all day. But when exercise is short and intensive it should be exhilarating, stimulating, fun and BRIEF.

So far I've only considered what I consider to be wrong with what actually happens at the average gym. What should also be thrown into the mix is what's missing from almost everybody's gym experience.

Well quite a lot actually. Let's see.

- ✗ *Balance and agility – I almost never see anyone doing anything balance related in the gym.*

- ✗ *Bodyweight work – being able to handle our own bodyweight well is a prerequisite for living well and performance in sport. I rarely see anyone do so much as a pull-up in a gym.*

- ✗ *Flexibility and posture – although gym programmes usually toss in a few stretches for good measure, these are usually inappropriate and never lead to long-term improvements in range of movement.*

✗ *A suitable dietary approach for weight-loss, health and better body composition – what can I say? Most gyms offer no advice, or simply echo the government's failed 'low-fat, healthy grains' approach.*

✗ *Confidence in challenging, three-dimensional movements which require concentration and improved coordination to perform. The body needs to be challenged in three different directions (forward and back, side to side, and rotationally) in order to develop as a whole unit.*

✗ *Support – it's called a 'health and fitness club' but, let's face it, there's nothing 'club-like' about it at all. It'll take months to get to know anyone and when they do speak to you it'll probably just be to check that you're finding it as fruitless a process as they are.*

I am going to finish this chapter by acknowledging that there are a few gyms out there that are not guilty of much of the above. They are few and far between, but if you can get to a **Crossfit gym** you'll do pretty well for yourself. They have few machines (although they are strangely fond of rowing) and rely on natural, three-dimensional movements that emphasise strength, power, balance, endurance and agility. Their workouts are very tough and rugged however. You can easily find yourself over-training in a place like this, but your efforts won't be wasted as they are in a conventional gym. Many also have an idea about good nutrition, and most actually want you to turn up as their business model isn't as cynical as the others'.

So Crossfit gyms get my stamp of approval, but otherwise I recommend that you give the gym a miss. If you love it, it's possible to use one sensibly, but most of the good stuff you could do at home, in the garden or in a park.

I've spent the whole of this chapter being very negative. Please be assured – there is light at the end of the tunnel!

Key Chapter Points

- *Regular gyms are not designed for you, but for bodybuilders with very specific aesthetic goals (which only work with extreme nutritional plans).*

- *Gyms primarily want your money, not your attendance. (It's their business model that most of their customers don't attend)*

- *Most gym equipment is hopeless for achieving the goals of ordinary people.*

- *Machines isolate muscle function, meaning there's very little transferral of ability to your own life. The best you might get is 'good at gym'.*

- *Cardio machines are a wasted opportunity to get outside and enjoy all the benefits that this brings. They are almost always used incorrectly, so that weight loss is harder and fitness gains are compromised. Overtraining is easy.*

- *Many of your basic fitness needs (three-dimensional balance, agility, power, co-ordination and real-world strength) will not be addressed by a conventional gym or the off-the-peg programme you'll be given.*

- *You're not alone if you dislike the atmosphere in your gym. It's a lonely, soulless place that doesn't fulfil your basic need for real movement.*

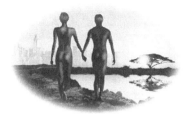

CHAPTER ELEVEN

Natural Living

"If our nature is allowed to guide our life,
we grow healthy, fruitful, and happy"

Abraham Maslow

In the previous chapters we have looked mostly at what might be considered the 'hard' skills of Instinctive Fitness: the 'nitty-gritty' nuts and bolts of how to get your *body* into better shape.

This chapter is about taking a more rounded view: the 'soft' skills for a great life if you like. Right back at the beginning of the book I claimed that Instinctive Fitness is not just another diet or exercise routine, and indeed it isn't. In this chapter I'd like to discuss how you can adopt a whole new lifestyle philosophy towards your own wellbeing and that of those around you.

This book has already suggested some new behaviours for getting your *body* in shape, but lifelong health involves more than just a good approach towards food and exercise. Feeling totally happy in yourself is perhaps only 50% about physical looks and performance, with the other half coming from having a relaxed outlook without undue stress.

> Our existence is nothing more than one big game: a game we're all going to ultimately lose sooner or later – so why not have a happy, playful, adventurous view on life while it is here?

Recap

The easiest, most instantly effective improvement you can make to put the spring back in your step is changing what you put in your mouth; it's an area of your life you should be able to control with relative ease once you better understand those instincts! The food you choose to eat really can make an instant difference to how you look, feel and perform. Try it and see!

Movement, we have already covered at some length too; so this chapter attempts to outline other important factors that are not strictly about the body, but on which a truly happy, healthy life also depend.

Embracing a more natural existence

I do believe that there are certain ways of living that are in harmony with our own nature as human animals. Where our lives deviate from the blueprint our genes expect, we set ourselves up to a greater or lesser extent for discomfort, disease and unhappiness.

Let's consider what sort of positive triggers our bodies expect to engage with. Beyond proper nutrition and regular movement, our genes expect a number of *other* things.

The following factors I consider to be broadly **physical:**

- *Adequate rest and sleep*
- *Exposure to sunshine and outdoor life*

The following points are largely sociological or **psychological;** essentially they are strategies to combat the biggest life wrecker and killer of all: long-term uncontrolled **STRESS:**

- *Physical challenge and meaningful risk*
- *Play and festivity*
- *Love*

Stress: the silent killer

Our stress response is natural and is there to give us a 'turbo boost' button when we need it most, and without a massively powerful reaction to moments of stress, ancient man would never have survived to pass on his genes to us.

During times of immediate danger from predators or during the excitement of the hunt they would have experienced what today would be called 'extreme stress': times when the 'fight or flight' mechanism is triggered. This response to stressful situations today enables us, just like our ancient ancestors, to reach new heights of performance – both physically and mentally. In times of high adrenalin the human body can perform at a higher level than normal and is capable of feats simply not possible in day-to-day life.

In a previous life my co-author was a fire-fighter and has experienced this adrenalin-fuelled 'high' many times. He once put the challenge to me to pick a fully grown adult up from a seated position on the ground by lifting them under their arms with my hands – not a chance, and nor can he normally! But in the line of duty, when the chips were down and with his body on high alert, he has done this many times without ever straining.

Stress and adrenalin are invaluable and essential in short bursts when required, but *lethal* when inadvertently left switched on for months or even years.

Our cosy modern world leaves us few opportunities to unleash our fight or flight instincts and crank our bodies up to the max. But our ancient bodies *yearn* to release these hormones from time to time to stay healthy. Today with few dangers or 'chases' to perform, our stress response hormones 'leak' uncontrollably into our bloodstream.

It is accepted in modern medicine that stress is a key factor in many medical conditions and diseases. The ability to release these natural hormones in a controlled way through physical play and by indulging in intrinsically relaxing activities can reduce stress levels naturally without resorting to drugs.

Managing Stress

With Instinctive Fitness, as for our hunter-gatherer ancestors, fitness, vitality and potency are not the *intention* of the lifestyles we lead; they are a by-product. Exercise is not a goal that needs to be clawed for, but is just time for physical play. A paleo diet is not eaten just to make us look a certain way – it's because frankly it tastes better without the 'claggy' starch-filled products and is more nourishing. Eating and exercise should both be enjoyable; activities should be looked forward to; and if it hurts or is uncomfortable - you're doing something wrong!

> Instinctive Fitness is about daring to be more playful in your whole outlook on life; in the activities you participate in, in the food you cook and in the way you interact with other people.

We believe that in having a more relaxed attitude toward the quest for health and fitness, and a playful attitude towards life as a whole, both mental and physical mastery will come along all by itself without much conscious effort.

On a long-term basis, thinking too much and fretting about exercise and nutrition can in itself produce stress. Adrenaline has a corrosive long-term effect on the whole body – like a raucous, out of control party, it's exciting, exhilarating, and fun for an evening, but is not likely to do you, your health or your bank account a lot of favours if protracted over weeks or months.

The irony of this is that many of us seek the buzz of constantly high adrenaline levels, pursuing pseudo high octane activities like consoles games, movies, gambling or internet surfing. Any of these activities in short bursts is arguably a good release of stress, but all too often the rush of adrenaline becomes an addiction and can become all-consuming to the point of obsession. Adrenalin continuously pumping around the system is not good for the body and can result in an addiction to the activity itself.

> Any area of life where you just can't help yourself from over indulging, is one you should perhaps take a closer look at. Have your basic animal instincts been hijacked by modern hyper-stimuli beyond your control? Tread carefully!

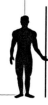

Most people in our information-saturated, break-neck modern world have lost the ability to hold complete focus on anything due to chronic levels of stress. They can only relax when distracted from their own feelings and immediate environment – hence why the most popular form of relaxation is drinking alcohol in front of the TV, which is a distraction from both ourselves and our situation.

The best tips for relaxation are to **slow down, do one thing at a time, and breathe evenly**. Relax your shoulder and neck muscles – if you can get your body to relax you'll soon find your mind follows. Too often we rush about, multi-tasking and worrying about stuff that may never happen.

Staying present

For our ancestors, staying alive meant that they had no option but to stay tuned to the present moment to sense possible danger. This meant that they could not afford to indulge in any tendency towards day-dreaming, introspection, over-analysis or worry. They were able to appreciate what they had rather than dwelling on what they did not.

Many of the world's religions emphasise stillness, gratitude and awareness, usually through prayer and meditation. It seems to me that in doing so, they are fulfilling our deepest instinctive need for a greater experience of the present moment and a more profound reverence for life and nature. These practices fulfil a modern desire to escape from our endlessly churning, critical, verbally-orientated mind, and to re-experience the sensation of observing life as it really happens.

Could it not actually be the calm, focused intensity and awareness of the hunter that is really missing in our lives?

An attitude of gratitude

Modern researchers into happiness and positive psychology repeatedly emphasise how important gratitude is in establishing a happy outlook. Being without the influence of a consumer society, our historic predecessors would not have felt they wanted for much while there was a steady supply of food about. They thanked their gods for favourable hunting outcomes and that increased their sense of gratitude and good fortune.

Today we are constantly bombarded with marketing messages from the media telling us what we *haven't* got and what we're *lacking*. It makes us feel in some someway *deficient* and that we could instantly feel more worthy if we just whipped out the credit card again.

To me, a focus on **gratitude** and **life as it happens** is the beginning of the enlightened life. Our modern western mind is dominated by analytical thought, self-absorption and a lack of spontaneity. It's also plagued with rampant consumerism, with the message being that we can never have enough.

"Work, work, work, buy, buy, buy" it tells us. Without meaning to, we end up working harder than we want to, to buy stuff we don't need, for spare time we don't have, with a family we may rarely see.

Is it going too far to say that the hunter-gatherer ethos offers an alternative mental, emotional and spiritual model, as well as a superior physical one?

Adequate rest and sleep

In the quest for physical fitness, rest is often overlooked as a factor. Rest represents your body's chance to remake itself anew. Physical improvement is usually predicated on some sort of process of breakdown when the body is challenged and works overtime to repair and improve. If we train hard or work hard and do not allow adequate time for recovery, overload is the result and any gains are quickly reversed.

Maerk's family left plenty of time for relaxing, having fun, playing and generally chilling out. They wouldn't have worked harder at the business of living than they had to – and yet today many people would look down upon this attitude; especially those addicted to their work. In contrast, Maerk and his family worked to live; they certainly didn't live to work!

Sleep

Before the advent of time pieces, humans went to sleep when they felt tired, which was usually not long after night-fall. The cyclic nature of the day means that our natural hormonal balance shifts towards encouraging sleep after sunset. Most of us (despite modern trends) do not function well on less than 8 hours sleep a day; short changing ourselves in this area is storing up long-term problems as well as short-term fatigue.

Most of the research on sleep points towards the idea that getting to bed early and rising with the sun is the most natural pattern to adopt. Interestingly, some research suggests that sleeping in two phases ('bi-phastically') might be the method most in line with our ancient history. This may have been an evolutionary adaptation that meant that there would always be someone awake (if only for an hour or two) during the night to watch out for the welfare of their snoozing companions.

From this I take away the message that if I awaken during the night after going to sleep 'too early', I shouldn't worry about it, but should instead enjoy the peace and solitude before returning for the second portion of my night's R&R.

I like to keep my bedroom quite cool and my bed pretty warm; I think I sleep better this way. I don't set an alarm clock, but I wake up naturally soon after day-break. If you've got things right you should wake up early, refreshed and ready to go. If you went to bed early enough and stayed there long enough, but still found you didn't get a good eight hours of sleep, then it's time to experiment.

One thing to look at straight away is whether you spent your final hours awake staring at a TV or computer. If you did, the strength of the light will be telling your body that it's still the middle of day; so when you plunge it into the darkness of your bedroom it is far from prepared for sleep.

Gradually creeping darkness encourages the body to release hormones that slow the body down and relax the mind, in preparation for slumber. If you must watch TV, watch it in the early evening, rather than just before bed. If possible, gradually dim the lights through the evening with the use of dimmer switches or even candles on the dinner table. Or maybe – even more authentically – rely on the flickering light from a log fire in the hearth?

It's easy to gloss over the sleep issue: "Okay so I don't sleep that well – so what?"

Poor sleep has a number of quite serious deleterious effects:

1. *It lowers our production of essential hormones like testosterone and growth hormone (which encourages the formation of adipose tissue through lower fat burning).*

2. *It maintains high stress levels (through higher levels of a hormone called cortisol) and therefore raises the risk of depression, high blood pressure and our susceptibility to diabetes and heart disease.*

3. *It reduces insulin sensitivity, meaning we handle the carbohydrates in our diet even less well, making it even harder to lose weight.*

When we sleep well, our immune system is strengthened, we lose fat, and physical and mental health improves.

So sleep well!

Exposure to Sunlight and the Outdoor Life

In common with all creatures, humans were born to live outdoors. We have known for some time that people who rarely see sunlight (perhaps because they live inside the Arctic circle in winter or, more likely, because they have an office job) suffer from low levels of Vitamin D. UVB rays from the sun interact with cholesterol in our skin to produce what is an essential hormone affecting the functioning of our whole body.

Moreover, the right amount of sunlight is essential for building stronger bones and fighting osteoporosis, assisting fat loss, raising testosterone levels, strengthening the immune system, reducing inflammatory conditions and improving psychological wellbeing.

SAD (Seasonal Affective Disorder) has been well documented as a phenomenon affecting those who see little sunlight during the winter months. It has been hypothesised that this may account for the unusually high numbers of suicides in Scandinavia, even though these countries enjoy the highest standards of living in the world. Summer holidays do more than just offer rest and change; they also allow us to top-up our Vitamin D levels and shift our hormonal balance in a favourable direction.

Avoiding sun burn to lower the risk of skin cancer is essential, but hiding from sunlight entirely and only venturing outdoors occasionally – and then only slathered in Factor 40 sun block – makes no sense at all. Only by regularly getting large areas of skin exposed to *moderate* levels of UVB light can your body function at its best.

In terms of the outdoor life, humans developed in various different environments, but all of them were natural rather than man-made. We are more relaxed and in-touch with ourselves in natural surroundings. Physical contact with nature and animals gives us a sense of reconnecting with something that is usually lost in the artificiality of urban life.

Recently, reports have emerged that while protecting the skin, sun cream with too high a factor may actually be *damaging* children's health. Rickets, a disease that makes bones malleable and which was once thought to have been banished from this country, is increasingly popping up again on the healthcare radar. Caused again by a lack of Vitamin D, rickets was common place in the smog-shrouded, sun-deprived cities of the 19th century. However, today, many parents will not let their children out without being smothered head to foot in factor 50 which reflects much of the sun's vitamin forming rays.

Our friend Maerk would surely have avoided getting burnt in the midday sun, but would have still enjoyed a year-round tan, built up slowly and carefully over a lifetime.

Take home message: you need nature and sunshine to thrive. Get away from urban life and enjoy sunshine in a natural environment when you can.

Physical challenge and meaningful risk

In a world increasingly obsessed with 'elf and safety', finding anything remotely risky to do when getting physical is not an easy task. When we were young (especially us boys) we liked to lay it all on the line when the opportunity arose: climbing a tall tree, venturing into a field with a bull, playing games we really shouldn't in derelict buildings – all just for the thrill.

Today as adults we've had *"Is it safe?"* hammered into us to the extent that our natural instinct to take a calculated risk for worthwhile reward has been all but squashed. We now get our 'kicks' cheaply and second-hand from films, television and video games.

All these imposters are designed to fire up the 'fight or flight' adrenalin kick we all so enjoy, and are our sterile and safe modern world's way of offering a cheap thrill without ever actually laying safety on the line. Yet we all yearn to be scared from time to time – why else would film studios rake in huge profits producing films that are frankly designed to do nothing else but scare the pants off us?

It should come as no surprise that the stars of sports such as Formula One, Moto GP and boxing are some of the best paid and most revered. Take the driver out of a racing car and control it remotely from the pits and it simply doesn't have the same allure. We love that our hero's prepared to pay the ultimate price for the glory, because at heart we ourselves would die for the same thrill.

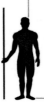

NASA never *needed* to send a man to the moon to achieve its scientific objectives. But NASA did need to pay for all the fun and games it was planning. To do that, it needed money – and lots of it. The only way to persuade the taxpayers of America to stump up the *billions* of dollars required to get them into space was to sell the general public a dream; so they captured their imagination by offering up modern day gladiators – heroes prepared to risk it all on top of a 111 meter high, 129 tonne 15,700 mph bomb.

Instinctive Fitness isn't about being shot at the moon or even climbing up the outside of a tower block without a rope; it's not about taking foolish risks just for a kick, but it is about pushing your mental and physical limits.

Risk and reward activities – not exercise

Any physical activity undertaken with the true spirit of Instinctive Fitness involves not only some sort of movement but a challenge: an element of risk and reward that is controlled and exciting rather than laborious or dangerous.

- *How about the 'rush' of sprinting down a steep hill faster than you feel comfortable – risking a tumble?*

- *How about pull ups hanging from a foot bridge above a small stream – no danger but the very real risk of getting cold and wet.*

- *What about a game of paintball with a sizable forfeit – imagine the intensity of the experience when the consequences of being hit are cleaning the victor's car inside and out!*

Instinctive training should have, wherever possible, an element of risk/ reward and exhilaration, although in reality not any real danger. Any form of exercise should leave you feeling better than before you started. Not just because it's a better way of gaining any fitness goals you may have, but because we want our brain to keep dragging us back – associating exercise with pleasure not pain.

There are many other activities that are great for enjoying in themselves *and* provide fantastic fitness benefits. Obviously, unless you're very rich and have plenty of 'play time', some of these are unlikely to form part of your *daily* activities but, should you get the chance, they fall right into the IF ethos.

tree climbing	*bouldering*	*surfing*
skateboarding	*martial arts*	*white water canoeing*
paintballing	*'capture the flag'*	*paddle boarding*
mountain biking	*rock jumping*	*teasing crocodiles.*
wild swimming	*friendly wrestling*	
go-cart racing	*free-running*	

I was just kidding with the last one – but you get the point.

The Fight or Flight Experience

Obviously it's not wise to replicate the conditions that set off a *true* fight or flight mechanism just for training's sake. However, by playing a psychological game, 'Fight or Flight' training actually replicates the exhilaration and heightened physical response called for in times of crisis.

We believe that allowing the body to run at its *real* maximum capacity for just a minute or two at a time provides a host of health benefits over the long term. Giving the adrenal gland the chance to switch into full flow and giving the body a chance to operate at flat-out maximum enables the adrenalin to shut off completely when we don't need it, and allows the body to relax properly afterwards.

Check out www.instinctive-fitness.com for more ideas on great ways to have fun while unintentionally getting fit.

Play and festivity

Although hunter-gatherers endured some tough times, these were matched by plenty of time for play, fun and relaxation. The natural way to celebrate a big kill was with a big feast. When they overcame genuine challenges (rather than the artificial type we know today, like 'surviving' an internal audit), their relief was easily expressed in dancing, joy, festivity and rest.

Today, many of us struggle to exert ourselves, even once a week – and yet find it harder still to truly relax when we want to. Tension and a feeling of dissatisfaction are almost endemic in our world where we are neither fully physically challenged nor truly at rest. We need this Yin and Yang to enable us both to 'switch on' fully and to 'switch off' fully. This middle ground malaise is quite simply sabotaging our time to recharge, lose our self-consciousness and truly celebrate just *being*.

Our lives are becoming increasingly regimented, ordered, measured and made to march to a timetable. Try adding more opportunities for just messing about, exploring, having fun, and generally just being playful.

(Climb a tree, put on a play with your kids, write a poem, chase your dog in circles – it doesn't matter much). Spontaneous playfulness is at the heart of creativity; it's the spark of genius at the centre of both our social and working lives - if only we could just stop being so uptight about productivity and tap its creative energy.

Living a natural life isn't just in the details – it's in the spirit. Loosen up a bit. Get out and do things; experience things. Spend less time worrying about being able to afford stuff. What you can't afford is to miss this precious time you have alive. Relax and enjoy what you have. Appreciate the good things and the good people you already have in your life.

Love (and loyalty and support)

At the risk of sounding a bit soppy, I'll remind you that Abraham Maslow (the best known positive psychologist of all time) considered love to be a central tenet in his famous hierarchy of human needs. (By now you'll have noticed that I love anything in a pyramid!)

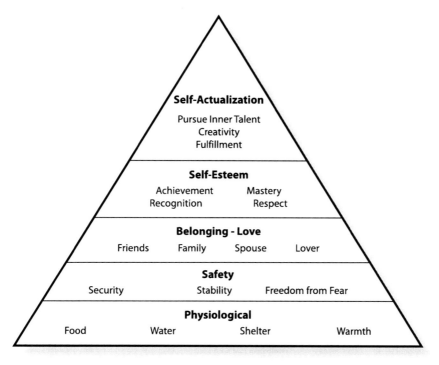

In a very real sense we can say that every human needs love. (The Beatles, of course, were right when they sang: "All you need is love!") Going back thousands of years, *every* human could expect love, cherishing, and validation; a sense of identity provided by their tribe, family and chosen partner.

They lived in an era when each and every day they could prove their worth and from their actions they knew their place in the order of things. These days, with our fractured sense of tribal loyalty (I don't think being a Manchester United fan counts), our divided families (divided by geography, attitude and generations) and our frequently single status (with divorce rates higher than ever), a sense of belonging is increasingly rare – however, it is, was and always will be a very special thing indeed.

For our ancestors, to be without any sort of love was to die; to be cast out of the tribe to wander until dead. Nowadays our fate may not be sealed in the same way, but a need to be cherished, approved of and appreciated never leaves us, no matter how grown up we might think ourselves. A life without love is one without meaning or direction. It descends to a basic level of fulfilling desires, characterised by shallow, selfish thinking and growing disillusion.

If you feel I am getting off-point on this thread, it's worth pointing out that since we appeared on this little planet pretty much the one subject that there *is* a consensus on from all purveyors of wisdom is that positive, balanced emotions are the backbone of good health, and that corrosive stressful emotions, such as loneliness, anger and sadness, are linked to weaker immune systems and a higher chance of developing serious illnesses.

Life is short and offers us but a small window of opportunity to feast on all its glories. Don't spend the years you *do* have worrying, stressing and feeling fearful. Seize the day! Every day, think and do nurturing things and the rewards of health, fitness and happiness will offer themselves willingly.

Chapter summary

- *Sleep well – it matters. Get your 8 hours or whatever your body needs. Get your body-clock back in line with the sun.*

- *Take time to relax in the evenings and at moments through the day.*

- *Get more sunshine (but don't get burnt!).*

- *Take on sensible physical challenges and meet them with awareness and present-moment focus.*

- *Stop stressing about things in the future which will never happen.*

- *Include time for fun, celebration and playfulness. There should be a time to have fun and be silly – it's a serious matter! Try exercising in a playful manner.*

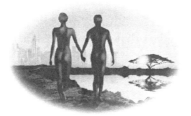

CHAPTER TWELVE

Putting it all together

"Knowing is not enough, we must apply.
Willing is not enough, we must do."

Bruce Lee

Just to recap, I consider there to be three main pillars which you should address if you are looking to completely overhaul your physical condition:

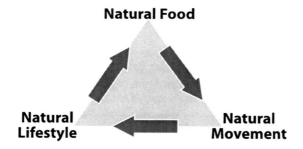

I will look at each one in turn and aim to show how you can gain the most benefits to be had from each with the least expenditure of effort. To use an ugly American phrase, I'll show you how to get the most 'bang for your buck'. What I will lay down for you is a path that will be suitable for most people, most of the time. If you are an international rugby star or have difficulties walking then these approaches may not be optimal, but the principles will still hold true.

Change your eating style: Eat Natural Food

Changing the way you eat is more powerful than any other single change you can make. Of the pillars that supports this programme, it is by far the most important.

Here's how I suggest you do it:

1. Clear your cupboards

If I was a food fascist I would have you go through all the food in the house and chuck out everything that doesn't have a place in the following food triangle. But I'm more pragmatic than that and will give you a whole week to get your kitchen in order:

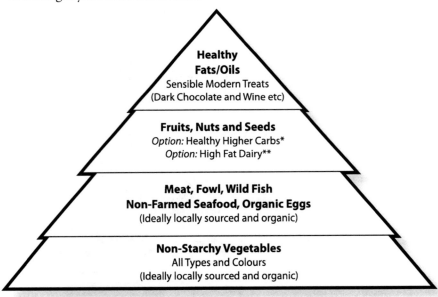

**Healthy
Fats/Oils**
Sensible Modern Treats
(Dark Chocolate and Wine etc)

Fruits, Nuts and Seeds
Option: Healthy Higher Carbs*
Option: High Fat Dairy**

**Meat, Fowl, Wild Fish
Non-Farmed Seafood, Organic Eggs**
(Ideally locally sourced and organic)

Non-Starchy Vegetables
All Types and Colours
(Ideally locally sourced and organic)

* e.g. sweet potato, wild rice, buckwheat – good, if not looking to lose weight)

** Be sure to do the withdrawal test to ensure dairy works with your digestive system.

The pyramid is arranged by recommended food *volume* (not calories, which would place meat, fowl, etc at the bottom instead of vegetables). The idea is that you eat more of those foods at the 'base' of the pyramid than those at the top.

This means you will chuck out all processed-foods, vegetable oils (and products containing them), grains (cereals, breads, biscuits, pasta, etc.), starches (including potatoes), sugars, margarines, table salt, skimmed and semi-skimmed milk, pasteurised cheeses, beans, mayonnaise, jams, spreads, malt drinks, fizzy drinks, energy drinks and concentrated fruit juices.

Also, you can eBay the toaster; you won't be needing it anymore!

You will want a kitchen that contains at least an oven, a hob, a kettle, a microwave and maybe a grill and slow-cooker.

2. Put clean, fresh foods into your kitchen.

The next step is to go and hit the shops. Alternatively you can get great food delivered. However, if you want the *very best*, it's frankly not much use heading to the supermarket. Specialist farmers will deliver a higher standard of meat and veg (organic as well as grass-fed). If all this five-star dining is outside your financial reach, then you will do okay at Tesco, Waitrose, Sainsbury's or any of the other big supermarkets, but you will need to move through them like a racehorse wearing blinders, shopping wisely.

If you are using a supermarket you'll find that most of the aisles contain foods which, according to my definition, are just 'bait' foods - i.e. they look appealing, but actually aren't fully edible (because nature didn't provide them for our consumption). Luckily, supermarkets tend to put these products in the middle of the shop. Most of what you will want is concentrated around the periphery of the building.

You will want to hit the grocery section really hard for fruit and vegetables (don't stray into the bread section!) before making for the fresh or frozen meat section. When buying meat, look for a variety of different animal types (including fowl and game). Choose big joints, large racks of ribs, or other large portions. Buying in bulk like this will keep down both costs and time spent preparing foods, as I'll explain shortly. Always choose organic if you can afford it. (It's worth it, so consider your priorities!)

After that, you will want to choose some fresh or frozen fish, some frozen vegetables or berries (for convenience) and possibly pick up a few bottles of organic milk.

Next you'll need to find some 'healthy' fat for cooking. Look for lard, goose fat, butter (organic), coconut oil, ghee (hard to find) or other animal fat. Additionally, choose a high-quality extra virgin olive oil for salads.

If you need any flour for bulking up dishes, choose coconut flour, almond flour, or ground arrowroot (these are all unprocessed, ground products).

You'll also want to pick up some eggs and some bacon. High-end burgers and sausages can now also be found that are 100% beef and free from gluten (breadcrumbs), so these are okay too.

When you get home, you will find that these will mostly, being fresh products, need to go into the fridge or freezer. Freeze all of the meat apart from some bacon and whatever meat you will cook next. The more freezer space you have here the better. Only a few things, like herbs, will need cupboard space.

3. Plan ahead for every meal:

Evening meal (you'll see why I'm listing this first in a moment)

Choose a meal the whole family will enjoy. Take time to consider making something special. This is the most important meal; it's ideal if everyone is present and sits around the table. (If you don't socialise at meal times, when will you?) You should have defrosted your chosen meat (or fish) prior to the time you start to put the meal together.

Take time to check out a recipe book or just have fun improvising if you're a creative or carefree cook. Don't forget that your meal will need to be composed of about 2/3 vegetables and 1/3 meat/fish/eggs. (In terms of calories it's more like 40/60 though).

I'll suggest some meal options in a minute, but the important thing is to cook loads of meat, certainly more than your family can possibly eat at one sitting, and place it on a large platter in the middle of the table. Then let people help themselves to the meat and the veg, taking as much or as little as they want. It may be a bit of a culture shock if you're used to bringing portioned plates to the table, but here are the advantages:

- *Everyone has the chance to eat until they are full. No one leaves the table hungry.*

- *Nobody ends up eating more than they feel like just because the family custom is that all the food is finished.*

- *There is plenty of meat left over for at least a meal or two the next day, which means you save on cooking time. Simply jazz it up a bit and re-serve.*

- *It justifies buying large joints, which means you can buy meat more economically.*

We all do this 'cheat' at Christmas, so why not the rest of the year?

If you want to save even more kitchen time, *buy a slow cooker.* At lunchtime, get someone to chop up some vegetables and throw them into the pot, add lots of meat. Then leave it for 4-9 hours. The beauty of this is that food is ready to eat whenever you want it. You can then eat immediately when you get home in the evening if you wish. You don't have to be present while it cooks!

Another advantage of this is that if you can't all be present for supper (shame on you!), family members can serve themselves whenever it suits them.

Breakfast

This tends to be the meal most people struggle with because we are all so accustomed to reaching for a quick bowl of cereal, toast or croissant. Please, whatever you do, avoid carbs here! Instead, look to make something with eggs, fruit, fish, or light meats (an idea that Europeans find easy). You could even have a portion of traditional English minus the toast and hash browns! Tuck into eggs, either scrambled or fried in butter or lard; add some bacon, grilled mushrooms, grilled tomato, quality sausages, chicken liver – whatever you fancy. Perhaps you could have a plain omelette or something with tuna, or a simple fruit salad - or just dig back into some meat from last night's supper. With just a few extra minutes and a little bit of imagination you really can set your day off to a great start!

Lunch

This is your opportunity to get loads of flavoursome and nutrient-loaded vegetables inside you. It's also a chance to ensure you get a good supply of satiating protein and fat into your stomach. I recommend that you make a massive salad. Cut up every vegetable in sight and throw them into a salad bowl, then add some meat from last night's feast. Or you could fry up some fish quickly. Throw in a few nuts, seeds and some grapes. Add a dressing made of virgin olive oil, lemon juice and sea salt; add any other spices that take your fancy. If you don't eat it all, you can refrigerate it and use it as a side-salad for your evening meal.

At this point I'm often asked "What actual meals can I eat? Are there any meals that will excite me? I mean, what does that leave?"

Here's my non-exhaustive list as a response to that. Most of these might be considered 'suppers' (or 'dinners'), but they could just as easily be eaten for lunch as well if you have the time to prepare them.

Meal options and ideas

(Just add more veg!)

- *Hotpot (Chicken/lamb/pork)*
- *Curry with cauliflower rice*
- *Beef stir fry*
- *Roast chicken/beef/pork with roast vegetables*
- *Garlic lamb kebabs (on a stick) with veg*
- *Baked fish*
- *Grilled chops/fish/steak*
- *English breakfast – bacon, sausage, onion, mushroom, tomato*
- *BBQ chicken and salad*
- *Steamed halibut and veg*
- *Beef burgers (100% beef) with mixed frozen veg*
- *Meatballs and sautéed fresh tomatoes*
- *Chilli-con-carne with tomato*
- *Pork and apple casserole*
- *Lamb tagine*
- *Grilled beef heart with roasted peppers*
- *Curried salmon salad*
- *Crockpot pork-stuffed peppers*
- *Omelette with bacon*
- *Shrimp salad*
- *Rabbit and onion casserole*
- *Salt and pepper squid*
- *Aromatic whole grilled chicken*
- *Sesame chicken and "rice"*

- Shrimp, sausage and summer squash casserole
- Cajun style blackened chicken liver and lemon and garlic sauce
- Thai green curry
- Lobster, grapefruit and avocado salad
- Scrambled egg and smoked salmon
- Sausage casserole
- Bacon, chicken and avocado salad
- Tender beef tongue with onion and garlic
- Bacon, egg, tomato and avocado salad
- Pork tenderloin with cilantro pesto
- Medallions of lamb with spinach
- Beef goulash
- Garlic-pulled pork
- Zesty lemon-and-lime seafood salad
- Sushi
- Stir fry liver with courgettes
- Frittata aleta
- Arctic chowder
- Organic prawn curry
- Chicken and shrimp soup
- Watercress and bacon soup
- Beef stroganoff with deep-fried cauliflower
- Grilled spareribs with boiled asparagus
- Oxtail casserole with Brussels sprouts
- Peppered salmon steaks
- Stuffed marrow/butternut tomatoes/onion/squash – best with mince
- Kippers with avocado puree
- Tuna salad with broccoli
- Italian spinach flan with Brussels sprouts
- Steamed scampi
- Mushroom stuffed with lamb's kidney
- Pork escalope
- Salmon steak in red wine
- Kidneys in sherry sauce with stuffed peppers
- Oriental stir-fry with coconut sauce
- Tiger prawn curry and cauliflower rice
- Lobster/crab
- BBQ'd pork and green pepper brochettes
- Lamb offal with pureed carrots
- Baked herring
- Sausages, grilled, with mixed vegetables, steamed.
- Lamb casserole
- Summerset style pork
- Prawn and pear salad
- Chilli pork with leeks in red wine
- Thai stir-fried vegetables with meat of choice
- Curried aubergines
- Foil-baked bass
- Lamb ratatouille
- Tossed green salad with avocado

- *Red cabbage campagnard with bacon*
- *Sauerkraut (v. healthy but needs 4 weeks to ferment)*
- *Greek vegetable soup*

- *Liver pâté*
- *Chicken a la king*
- *Haddock/cod/salmon – instantly cookable in microwave with veg of choice*

For more recipe ideas, please visit www.instinctive-fitness.com/recipes

Free your palette

If you don't find much in the list that whets your appetite, then you're probably still addicted to the carbohydrates prevalent in your current diet. It needs re-educating. Given time you will come to notice the 'claggy', heavy texture of bread and other grain-based products, and you'll regain your instinct and taste for *real* food.

When transitioning to low-carb, it is possible to go too far, too soon. If you do, you will start to feel a **low-energy 'fug'** and possibly suffer from low-moods. Don't worry, it is only temporary and will probably only last a few weeks, but you can make the transition easier by allowing yourself some healthy carbs, such as wild rice, sweet potato, or quinoa, when you need them. However, if you overdo the carbs you'll not lose any weight, so be judicious. Ensuring you include more fat in your diet and not just extra protein is essential.

Obviously you also need to be careful in how you prepare these foods. You need to make these meals entirely at home (no microwave versions out of tin trays!) and you mustn't add banned ingredients! Try not to add corn flour to your dishes, for instance; instead use the alternative bulking ingredients already mentioned. Most of these meals are delicious, simple to make and have recipes freely available on the internet by Googling "Paleo recipes". Any recipes that are part of the Paleo health movement will be suitable for you. There are many on Marks Sisson's superlative website www.marksdailyapple.com. There are also lots more inspirational pictures of personal transformations based on this way of eating than I can possibly fit in this book.

If you're still not sure that you're eating the right way or you're worried you're not getting the weight-loss you want as fast as you would like (1-2 pounds a week is great progress, by the way), then there is a painless way to check you're on the right track.

Open an account with a website like www.fitday.com. Input all your details and, for two or three representative days, record every morsel of food that you eat after each meal. This isn't as hard as it may sound – drop down menus make it very easy. With this tool you will be able to see how much carbohydrate you're *really* ingesting.

I would suggest that you need to get this well below 200g a day for success. 150 grams would be perfect. If you drop much lower than this, this would indicate that you are not actually eating enough vegetables because, remember, these are still carbohydrates – just not densely packed ones.

Use a system like this to ensure you've got things about right and then, pretty quickly, you will develop a feeling for what's right for you and what isn't. At that point you can give up the task of data entry after each meal.

I promise, even though paleo-style eating may sound like a shock to the system, and perhaps, for those used to instant food, a bit of a faff to prepare, it really isn't. With just a bit of strategic preparation and a new philosophy behind it, this way of eating is easily worth the minor effort involved.

Movement

Let's have another look at the Instinctive Fitness exercise pyramid where the activities at the base represent the activities you should pursue most frequently; and those at the uppermost tip, the least.

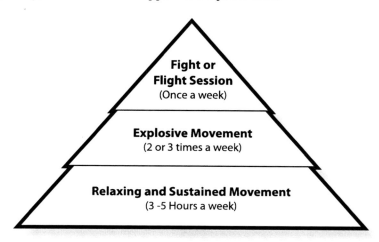

Outlined in the pyramid are suggested times you should commit to: what I call the **minimum effective dose.** Some people who really want to put in the effort could do rather more than this and get 20-30% fitter; however, the law of diminishing marginal returns kicks in quite quickly, so 'more' is optional depending on your lifestyle, goals and temperament.

You might like to make your week's activities look something like this:

Monday:	*Explosive movement* or heavy resistance task (12-25 mins)
Tuesday:	*Relaxed, sustained* walk (40 mins+) or rest if tired
Wednesday:	*Fight or Flight* session (15 mins, before or instead of low-carb breakfast)
Thursday:	*Relaxed, sustained* game of tennis, 9 holes of golf or walk (40 mins+) or rest if tired
Friday:	*Explosive movement* or heavy resistance task or strong resistance task (12-25 mins)
Saturday:	*Relaxed, sustained* 5 mile country/park walk (2 hours), or round of golf
Sunday:	Rest/play

This might look, from a distance, like an ordinary programme, but it's not. What's special about the above – and alternatives based around the same pyramid – is:

- *This programme doesn't have the one-sided bias towards any one single quality that most do. It's a programme for **total all-round development**. It's got all three of the different movement intensities we looked at in the Natural Movement chapter.*

- *The movements are all natural without any muscle group being isolated.*

- *The quantities are right – you won't burn out or fail to challenge yourself.*

- *There's plenty of recovery built in (3 days a week of rest if you need it)*

- *It's totally adaptable for what you like to do, your energy levels and your mood.*

- *It's enjoyable so you'll want to come back and do it again!*

Posture and good alignment

As we have previously discussed, posture and flexibility are the foundations upon which all the other areas of IF exercise are built. The type of exercise that Instinctive Fitness encourages in itself promotes good posture and flexibility. However let's run through a few areas you might like to look at to get you started.

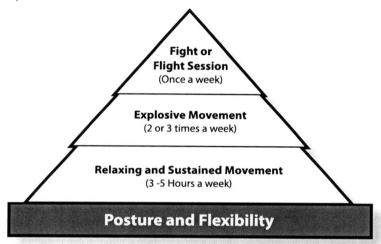

Posture is something that needs to be worked on constantly, but it doesn't actually require any specific time at all – just constant vigilance and awareness. You *will* need some help with this though – at least initially, until you are practicing the right way. To get onto the right lines, I advise you to purchase the book by Esther Gokhale called *"8 Steps to a Pain-free Back".* Esther's principles, instructions and pictures will soon have you on the way to a better posture and all-round improved performance. It is required reading for everyone from grandmothers to international athletes.

Buy it even if your back doesn't hurt now – if you follow her 8 steps it will change your life forever. Following her principles, built up over years of studying the postures of nations and cultures with no incidence of postural difficulties, is the single best thing you can do to guard against the ravages of old-age and spinal atrophy. I can't recommend it highly enough. If you're reading this in the UK, there are now teachers of her method here as well as in the USA.

Even if you don't buy the book, there's still plenty you can do to help yourself out:

- *Don't spend hours slumping in chairs*
- *Stand to work if you can (I am standing as I write this)*
- *Get up frequently to stretch and move about*
- *Take mini-breaks to get fresh air or march up and down the office stairs every 40 minutes or so*
- *Explore simple stretches, movements and mini-workouts you can do throughout the day in five-minute chunks*

Almost any movement will stop your discs totally compressing in the way they certainly will when sitting with your body in poor alignment; some exercises and stretches are much more effective than others though.

Two simple things you can do to improve your posture right now are to remember not to push your hips forward when you stand or to allow your tailbone to tuck under when you sit. Even in a seated position, your bottom should retain its distinctive 'bottom-like' shape. If it disappears when you sit, you're not doing yourself any postural favours.

Another idea – shoot me if you think this is terribly old-fashioned – is to place a bean bag on your head and balance it there while you go about your day. This is what African ladies have learned to do to maintain their exemplary posture, except that they tend to do it with enormous jars of water rather than with bean bags. Now don't get me wrong, I'm not suggesting you do this in the office or in public – you'll get funny looks – but in the privacy of your own home this little tip works pretty well. It stops you poking your head forward so much and pushing your hips forward. It also encourages better balance by encouraging you to glide rather than bounce up and down when you move.

As you become more aware of how you move around, try to get into the habit of hip-hinging when you bend for things. Learn to bend at the hips rather than in the back to pick things up. Don't bend your knees much unless you have to reach very low. Instead your hips should move backwards from their position over your feet in order for your upper body to become more horizontal.

Check out our website at *www.instinctive-fitness.com;* it's always being updated with new information on this sort of thing.

Sq- what?

The other essential movement that you need to work into your day more is the **squat**. This is a movement that our ancestors would have performed many times a day (especially when sitting around a fire). Include it in your workouts or use it in your mini-work breaks. Work up to the full squat by putting a 2" raised block under the heel of each foot. Mix them up by doing ordinary ones, wide ones, narrow ones, ones with your left foot forward, right foot forward and every combination in between. Then do it on uneven ground. You get the idea: variety is the key here. The increased strength and flexibility this will bring your legs and hips is extraordinary!

Walking

> *"Walking is the best exercise.*
> *Habituate yourself to walk very far"*

Thomas Jefferson

Walking gives us many of the same benefits as traditional aerobic activity (calorie burning, lowered blood pressure, lowered resting heart rate, lowered cholesterol, increased cardiac output, increased capillary density, increased nutrient/oxygen delivery, etc.) without all of the drawbacks (musculoskeletal injury, joint wear and tear, elevated stress hormones, muscle loss, lowered metabolic rate, etc.). Simply put, it's the aerobic activity we were born to do.

If you're going to be doing plenty of this then it makes sense to do it well. That means doing it as we evolved to. There could be a whole book on this subject, but a few basic principles will get you up and, er, walking.

Firstly footwear: even if you don't opt for the striking (read: 'eccentric looking') Vibram Fivefinger shoes I recommend, then at least ensure that your footwear has a thin soft-ish flat sole with plenty of room for your toes to spread. Avoid heavy shoes with any sort of elevated heel. A simple pair of gym shoes is still better for your health, poise and co-ordination than the best pair of Nikes. Just because you can't feel the impact of the road much in high-end trainers doesn't mean it's not there.

However, damage to your joints will accrue more slowly wearing cushioned shoes than if you carelessly slam your heels down in just the same way in paper-thin soles, so it's important that, like Maerk and his clan, you learn to tread softly and quietly again.

To encourage a natural stride, ensure that one foot is placed roughly in-line with the next, as if you were walking along a single white line. Having feet that run on two different tracks means that you lack balance and flexibility in your hips. Make sure you don't hold tension in your legs as you walk. If your head wobbles from side to side as you walk, or bounces up and down more than half-an-inch, you need to work on your technique and posture.

When you are walking well, you should feel your bum muscles contract as you take each step, rather than feeling the need to lift each foot and place it in front of you. Good walking should feel like it happens almost by itself.

Running

Good technique is hard to get a grip on until you can walk well, but upright balance is the key. Most of us hunker forward when we run, leading with our heads and tucking our pelvis under as we move. We tend to focus on pushing off with each long-stride rather than taking shorter-strides, cushioned by a little controlled bend in the knees.

If you really want to master this and run with the easy languid gait of a Kenyan miler or the effortless grace of Usain Bolt, I suggest you seek out a "Pose" running specialist near you. However if you work on your basic posture throughout the day, there will be some good transference to all your movements, including running technique.

The most essential principle is that your feet should be placed underneath you when running, not in front. Most people throw their feet out in front of themselves and then tumble forward on to them. They typically bounce up and down as they run and often sway from side to side too. This is wrong and is caused mainly by the harmful modern habit of heel-striking, which is only made possible by modern running shoes. (Yet another example of how modern technology has hindered more than helped!)

Heel-striking (landing on the heel and rolling forwards in each step) has only been possible since the advent of the cushioned running shoe 40 years ago and represents the single biggest cause of running injuries. Heels striking the ground in cushioned shoes (80% of runners) impact with *three times* the force of those habituated to barefoot running.[1] Is it any wonder that there are so many injuries these days?

A minimalist shoe is a good compromise, but slapping your heels down in a shoe that has no cushioning is a very quick way to injury. You need to get your form right, relearning how to run on the mid-foot or the balls of the feet with your body upright and your feet circling beneath you.

One of the quickest ways to improve running technique is to practice occasionally without any shoes at all. (This is the way you were born to run.) A slightly rough surface underfoot will soon have you cushioning every landing with the natural bend of your knees and the flexibility in the arch of your forefoot.

Having said that, if you transition to a minimalist shoe (or bare footing) too fast, and don't allow time for your softer foot-strike to catch up, you could end up injuring yourself. Be careful and get advice before embarking!

For more information on 'bare footing', see the work of Daniel Lieberman, Professor of Human Evolutionary Biology at Harvard University.

Four Sample Days of IF.

By outlining four days' worth of living I think I can give you a flavour how you can add food and exercise together while combining them with the other lifestyle suggestions I have made.

MONDAY:

Get up about 6am (after waking naturally with the sun). Drink a pint of filtered water. **25 mins explosive movement training.**

Breakfast Boil 6 eggs; eat 3 soft boiled with some spinach, salt and pepper to taste; hard boil the rest. *Take organic coffee if you like it. Mid-morning take a mini-work break – do as many different kinds of squats as you can think of. Do one or two of each - don't work up a sweat. Drink another pint of water before 10am.*

Lunch: Add the 3 hard-boiled eggs to a tuna salad, including mushrooms, onions, peppers, cucumber, broccoli, grapes, and plenty of greens. Add olive oil (and balsamic vinegar, if you like it.) *After lunch go for an 10 minute brisk walk outdoors and drink a pint of water afterwards. If hungry later, eat a handful of macadamia nuts.*

Supper: Cook a large roast chicken or joint of beef. Eat as much as you want with as much steamed cauliflower, courgette and carrot as you like. *Finish using the TV or computer before 8, and lower the lights for the rest of the evening. Be in bed by 9.45. Sleep when tired.*

TUESDAY:

Rise early for a **Relaxed, Sustained** walk (30 to 40 mins).

Breakfast: fruit-salad.

Lunch: Chicken (or beef) salad with last night's leftovers, using lots of romaine lettuce, cherry tomatoes, radishes, onion, bell peppers, avocado and various green vegetables. If you get hungry in the afternoon, try bottled olives as a snack, or have some more macadamia nuts. (Don't eat these if you're not hungry though).

Supper: None – just skip it and go to bed a little earlier. If you're new to this way of eating maybe hold off on this little fast until the rest of the programme is second-nature. *Other details the same as in the italics above.*

WEDNESDAY:

8 minute **Fight or Flight** session (using Tabata protocol - plus 5 min warm-up, 5 min warm down) on bicycle or on foot. Consider doing this barefoot if you can find a good stretch of ground.

Breakfast: Eat this as late as possible or just have a bigger-than-usual, early lunch. Choose scrambled egg, bacon and asparagus, or omelette and veg.

Lunch: Eat prawn salad with loads of veggies. Chop up extra vegetables and throw them into a slow cooker; add lots of lamb and cook on slow, ready for tonight's supper.

Supper: Eat your lamb casserole, with some fruit for 'sweet'. Make sure you eat until you're full. *Don't forget the italicised details above!*

(Tonight, after your fasted exercise and then the two good meals, your metabolism will be at racing speed. Ideal for fat burning!)

THURSDAY:

Breakfast: Eat a light breakfast of nuts, fruits and seeds with a little cream.

Lunch: Steamed fish (wild salmon maybe) and 2 or 3 veg (also steamed.)

Do something *fun* today; *play* a friendly game of tennis or squash; or have a kick-around in a park with your kids. Be sure to take it easy.

Supper: Stuffed butternut squash with mince or a huge rack of ribs (with plenty left over for tomorrow's lunch); add 2 vegetables of your choice. Take blueberries and a little cream for 'sweet', or a piece of fruit.

Motivation and attitude

It's important to approach this new healthier way of living with the right attitude. To start with, be kind to yourself. You weren't perfect before, and you're not likely to be perfect now. But you are going to do considerably better for yourself, and for your family too if they join you on this challenge. Remember that any change is tricky and you need to see it as a huge opportunity to gain something, not as a way to feel bad about yourself when you slip up. It's a journey; an adventure. It should be fun.

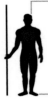

You're going to wander from the path, but it's not the end of the world. Don't be too tough on yourself. When you go wrong, you go wrong – all that matters is how quickly you get back on track.

I am not going to ask you to aim for anything less than 100% perfect, but I want you to allow yourself to score as low as 80% some days, or some weeks and still accept your efforts. You will still gain most of the promised benefits if you get things 80% right. (This is sometimes known as the '80/20 rule.') You can't mess things up very much with one or two bad meals a week or a day or two of sedentary living. It's the larger patterns that matter. How many days of good exercise did you fit in *this month*? How many non-processed meals did you manage to consume *this month*? This is the scale on which you can start to see the clear results of your efforts.

Please remember that this programme isn't a quick-fix system, or a short-cut to anything. Ultimately, there are no short-cuts to anything, no matter what the adverts tell you. Short-cuts in health terms are bad and tend to only give the illusion of progress. If you want to lose 21 pounds this month, it's easy. Just eat cabbage soup and nothing else. You'll get ill – but you'll have lost 21 pounds. If you want sustainable low-fat levels and high levels of health for the rest of your life – well that's different.

Take a long-term approach – and this is it. Nothing else is congruent with the bodies and genetics we have all been given. Remember that it's just a programme based around principles and our knowledge of our ancient past, *not* a cult, a fad or religion.

That's the key to it really: remember the WHY. Remember why you're doing this. Imagine in pictures the benefits you will enjoy in a month, a year, even ten years' time. Remember also WHY this is the programme that will work for you if you stick with it and trust in the process.

If you don't get the results you're hoping for fast enough, ask yourself the following:

- **Am I expecting too much too soon?** *Is it realistic to expect to lose all the fat around your belly while you still have plenty on your arms, for example? This programme isn't a magic bullet for overnight transformation. It is, however, the only programme I know that people can stick with and that will continue to pay dividends for years. You will overtake your friends on their yo-yo diets, but not because this programme works faster (it might not do) but because it will keep giving when they have long since quit. It will also be much healthier than their approach.*

- **Am I actually following the principles properly?** *How similar are most of your days to the four example days described above? Or have you got lots of little rationalised cheats going in your mind: "Well potatoes are vegetables aren't they, and if I fry them in coconut oil…"*

- **Am I expecting linear improvements?** *Life tends not to work like this. Nobody loses exactly 2 pounds a week for 5 months. Your body is much too complicated to be able to affect in such a predictable manner Some of my clients have lost no weight at all for the first few weeks. Before that though, most started enjoying superior levels of energy and lost two or three inches of grain-bloating around the waist.*

One thing you can do to help your progress is to journalise it. You could do this in a diary next to your bed, or start a blog to update supportive friends. One reason to do this is that it's human nature to forget quickly how much we've achieved and where we started from. Write down all your basic measurements and some performance benchmarks (press-ups, pull-ups, and squats – that kind of thing.)

These things are not the *reasons* for eating and living a more natural lifestyle, but they do tend to keep us on track. Just telling others about our intentions and any results can keep us accountable.

Having said that, others will fear you're gaining something that they haven't got the self-discipline or the know-how for, so don't be surprised when someone close tries to undermine your efforts. Expect the brainwashed low-fat crowd to scoff if you disclose affection for bacon, butter or full-fat organic milk.

Let your results speak for themselves!

When you reach mile stones (e.g. one month without grain), why not reward yourself with a something special to reinforce your achievement? (No, not a large Domino's Pizza!)

It's really important that, without departing from any crucial principles, you find ways to *enjoy the process* of turning things around. Find things that work for <u>you</u>: easy and delicious meals, enjoyable exercises, fun games and sports – that kind of thing. Personalise the programme as much as you can, focusing on the process and not just results.

Banish any images of what you *should* look like from your mind. Ignore the siren-call of the media for enormous muscles or a wispy figure; that's not always written on the genetic cards we were handed at birth. You can still look great with a bigger than average frame if you're a lady, or with the lean musculature of a Thai-fighter if you're a smaller than average guy. Sometimes learning to feel good about yourself is of greater importance than any possible aesthetic result you might achieve.

Remember also how much more there is to this than a concern with aesthetics. What about living longer? What about staying mobile into your 90s? What about attaining super-charged levels of energy? What about beautiful poise and a pain-free body. This is the meat and bones of Instinctive Fitness!

This book has not meant to lecture or impose an opinion on you; instead it was intended to offer you a completely new version of the truth. Instinctive Fitness is about making subtle as well as broad changes that will bring you closer in line with the instincts that nature gave you. Every change you make realigns you with the drives that worked so well for our forefathers, the only species of Hominid to survive the ruthless race of evolution (well, thus far!).

Here again are those instincts we met at the start of the book and what we can do with each to re-sculpture our bodies and re-launch our lives anew:

Working <u>With</u> Your Instincts

Put on weight whenever possible: *If you eat the Instinctive Fitness way, eating a high-fat, medium protein, low-carb diet, you'll find putting on weight will actually be difficult. If you start skipping meals for the sake of convenience, it's possible that you may have to guard against being too thin, just like our ancient ancestors did. However, with plenty of protein in your diet and some explosive movement, new weight will come in the form of muscle, rather than fat. Additional muscle burns fat through the day and is one of your best defences against frailty and ill health throughout life. Also, well-toned men and women are more attractive and more capable in every way.*

Crave sweet, salty and fatty foods: *Retrain your taste buds by eating the foods our instincts evolved to direct us towards. Fulfil your appetite for these tastes through a naturally high-fat diet based around meat, fish, fowl, fruit, seeds, nuts and veg. Re-sensitise yourself to the subtler tastes of good, natural food. When your palate recovers and your brain forgets about the hyper-stimulation it once received from shiny, packeted 'bait' foods and other food imposters, you will lose your cravings and your food addictions, you'll lose fat, and your blood sugar levels will stabilise, providing you with on-tap energy throughout the whole day.*

Rest whenever possible: *Build physical tasks into your day so that it's impossible to rest all day long. Ensure you include some explosive movement, maybe using a simple, brief workout routine similar to the one I outlined earlier in the book. Find active things to do that you enjoy doing. Learn to play and have fun with movement as you used to as a child. Make resting all day impossible, simply because it's just not your customary habit and not the way you chose to live. Do ensure that you include plenty of rest, however; avoid excess stress and refrain from overly intensive cardio routines.*

Eat whatever's available and tastes good: *Buy only pure, natural foods; not foods that have been messed about with in factories and undergone heavy processing. If the supermarket is filled with temptations for you, avoid it, shop elsewhere or shop online. Clear your* *cupboards of all the junk. Once you're surrounded by real food, you can feel free to eat until you're full and have a really good feast whenever you feel like it. Because your body knows that it is always well provided for, it won't feel the need to store those calories as fat.*

Eat whatever looks shiny, bright and healthy: *Learn to see the product itself. Don't be fooled by shiny packaging and the efforts of the media and advertising to hook your interest. Learn to read ingredients labels, particularly looking out for those danger ingredients: vegetable oil, sugar, sweeteners, etc. Ask yourself, is this food part of a natural eco-chain, or is it just 'bait' laid out to trap my well-meaning instinct?*

Wake up when it's light and sleep when it's dark: *Go to bed when you first start to get tired between 9-11pm. Sleep with the curtains open and wake up slowly and naturally as the morning light streams into your bedroom. Avoid excessive time spent in front of a screen as this will affect your ability to sleep deeply and wake rested.*

Copy the posture and movement of these around us: *Look for better role models – like some athletes and non-westerners who still move with the grace and poise that we all should.*

Finally, once you've found your feet don't forget your duty to spread the word. For too long we've been at the mercy of bad advice from government health advisors, from an ignorant media and from scientists stuck in dogmatic cul-de-sacs.

In evolutionary and genetic terms we are perfect; in environmental terms and behavioural terms we have seriously handicapped ourselves. Only when enough people are willing to think for themselves and kick against the boards will the balance tip. Then we can create a new generation of people who are free to enjoy all the blessings that form our inheritance if we only had the instinct and the wisdom to see it.

That's it then; all you need. However some readers will prefer reading about this than actually taking action. I am always frustrated by clients who find excuses and fail to take the first step to turn their lives around. Those that do, usually say one of a few things.

Sorry excuses I've heard a lot...

1. "I don't have time"

You don't have enough time on the planet *not* to make these changes. Everybody has the same amount of time in the day as the next person; what they lack is priority. If they choose not to implement these changes, then fine – but be honest and say "It's not that important to me". The approach I've outlined here is based on the 'minimal effective dose' idea: how to get the most out of the smallest investment in your time.

2. "I don't have the money"

Much of what's in this programme is free. You don't need a gym subscription. You don't need to buy any equipment unless you choose to. You don't need special supplements. You will be saving money on gym memberships, medical bills and overpriced, starch-filled 'peasant food' with no nutritional value. I will concede that your meat and vegetable bill might go up but, having said that, I can't think of a more important thing to invest in than your future health and happiness. Health is wealth, as the saying goes. Of the many areas in your life where you can save money, why choose your own wellbeing?

3. "I haven't got the self-discipline and it seems a bit complicated."

To me it seems simple, but it's part of my nature now; habit has made it easy. I agree, though, that any change can be difficult in the early days. I would encourage you to get help if you can. If you're organised you can make the changes and feel benefits pretty quickly, so ask for support from a personal trainer, a partner, friends – anybody who understands fully what you're up to. With my own clients I can organise everything for them – the weekly food ordering, the weekly meal plan, and the daily exercise schedule – so that it's as easy as it possibly can be. I've organised my 30-day free IF programme in just the same way. Just sign-up on the website: www.instinctive-fitness.com

4. "I'm not convinced it will work. What if it doesn't?"

Well what will you have you lost? Now compare this loss with the almost guaranteed loss of health and mobility that you face if you do nothing. Make your best choice and act now! The only way to know is to try. Every few hours that passes after you put this book down means that you're more likely to fall back into the modern, faddish habits that have got you to where you are now.

5. "I'll do this – it does make sense. Just not now. Next month will be better when…"

Most people believe they should wait for conditions to be right before they act. This attitude doesn't work. Ever. The one that does is "Do what you can, now!" The conditions will never be perfect, no matter how long you wait. If you can't face taking action right now, at least commit to learn more, read more; find out the truth behind the issues this book has presented. Perhaps just download our Free 30 day challenge from www.instinctive-fitness.com and see how easy it really is.

A final thought

As you sit here and absorb these last few words, considering whether to act now or to consign these pages back to the bookshelf, you might be wondering whether it's all true? Will it really make a difference to your life? Maybe you'll fail, as you might have done in the past when trying to make changes for the better.

Worrying, wondering and fretting about what's gone before and what will follow won't change the decision you must make at this moment. Are you going to grab your future with both hands and regain control of the animal instincts that served your ancestors so well?

Eat like a king once more, play like a child and live your life to the full. Take a leap of faith, return to your instincts and unleash your fitter, stronger and happier caveman within.

References:

1. Daniel E. Lieberman et al. (2010) "Foot strike patterns and collision forces in habitually barefoot versus shod runners." Nature 463, 531-535

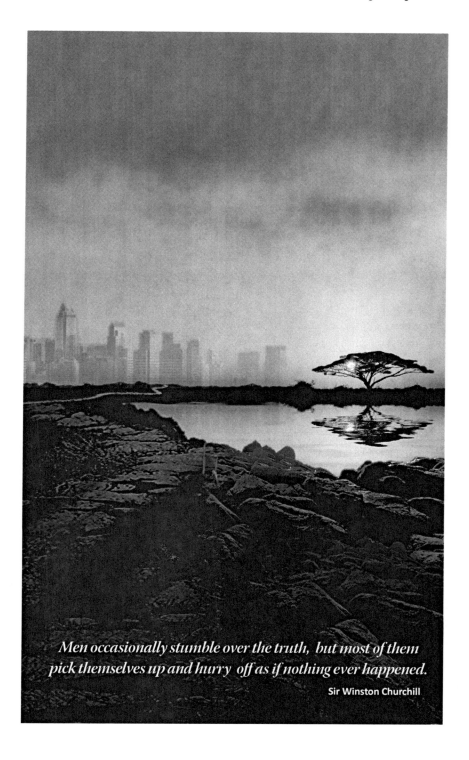

Men occasionally stumble over the truth, but most of them pick themselves up and hurry off as if nothing ever happened.

Sir Winston Churchill

About the Author

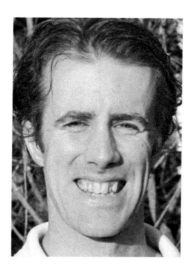

Oliver, 36, is a Personal Trainer from Oxford who
specialises in Mid-Life Body Transformations.
He gave up his job in journalism to retrain and
change people's lives after transforming his own
body and health with a system that confounds the
advice of conventional trainers and gyms.
He wrote Instinctive Fitness to let people
struggling to stay slim, healthy and energetic
know that there is a better way than stress,
striving and usually failing.

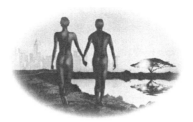

Bibliography

Academic

The Descent of Man by Charles Darwin and Michael T. Ghiselin *(Jan 14, 2010)*

Man the Hunter by Irven Devore and Richard B. Lee *(Dec 31, 1999)*

Limited Wants, Unlimited Means: A Reader On Hunter-Gatherer Economics And The Environment by John Gowdy *(Dec 1, 1997)*

First Farmers: The Origins of Agricultural Societies by Peter S. Bellwood *(Dec 6, 2004)*

Catching Fire: How Cooking Made Us Human by Richard W. Wrangham *(Sep 7, 2010)*

Evolution and Prehistory: The Human Challenge by William A. Haviland, etc. *(Mar 5, 2010)*

The Lost World of the Kalahari by Laurens Van Der Post *(Nov 3, 1977)*

Primitive Man & His Food by Arnold De Vries *(1900)*

Myth and Meaning: Cracking the Code of Culture by Claude Levi-Strauss *(Mar 14, 1995)*

Guns, Germs, and Steel: The Fates of Human Societies by Jared Diamond *(Jul 11, 2005)*

Lucy's Child the Discovery of a Human Ancestor by Donald C. Johanson *(Oct 31, 1991)*

African Archaeology: A Critical Introduction (Blackwell Studies in Global Archaeology) by Ann Brower Stahl *(Oct 4, 2004)* (Blackwell Studies in Global Archaeology)

The World of Primitive Man by Paul Radin and Stanley Diamond *(1971)*

Anthropology and Contemporary Human Problems by John H. Bodley *(Nov 9, 2007)*

Against Civilization: Readings and Reflections by John Zerzan *(May 10, 2005)*

Food and Western Disease: Health and nutrition from an evolutionary perspective by Staffan Lindeberg

The Omnivore's Dilemma: A Natural History of Four Meals by Michael Pollan *(Aug 28, 2007)*

Popular Science

The Primal Blueprint: Reprogram your genes for effortless weight loss, vibrant health, and boundless energy by Mark Sisson *(Jan 14, 2012)*

Beyond Broccoli: Creating a Biologically Balanced Diet When a Vegetarian Diet Doesn't Work by Susan Schenck Lac and Bob Avery *(Aug 20, 2011)*

The Paleo Answer: 7 Days to Lose Weight, Feel Great, Stay Young by Loren Cordain *(Dec 20, 2011)*

The New Evolution Diet: What Our Paleolithic Ancestors Can Teach Us about Weight Loss, Fitness, and Aging by Arthur De Vany and Nassim Nicholas Taleb *(Dec 20, 2011)*

8 Steps to a Pain-Free Back: Natural Posture Solutions for Pain in the Back, Neck, Shoulder, Hip, Knee, and Foot by Esther Gokhale and Susan Adams *(Apr 1, 2008)*

The Paleo Solution: The Original Human Diet by Robb Wolf and Loren Cordain Ph.D. *(Sep 14, 2010)*

Food Inc.: How Industrial Food is Making Us Sicker, Fatter, and Poorer-And What You Can Do About It by Participant Media and Karl Weber *(May 5, 2009)*

Good Calories, Bad Calories: Fats, Carbs, and the Controversial Science of Diet and Health by Gary Taubes *(23 Sep 2008)*

The Great Cholesterol Con by Dr Malcolm Kendrick *(7 Jul 2008)*

Wheat Belly: Lose the Wheat, Lose the Weight, and Find Your Path Back to Health by William Davis *(Aug 30, 2011)*

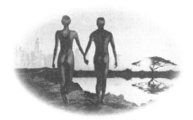

Websites:

http://www.health-report.co.uk/saturated_fats_health_benefits.htm

http://www.marksdailyapple.com/life-expectancy-hunter-gatherer/#axzz1ka7zRC14

http://beyondveg.com/billings-t/comp-anat/comp-anat-8b.shtml

http://www.proteinpower.com/drmike/

http://vimeo.com/ancestralhealthsymposium/videos

http://egwellness.com/what-hurts/lower-back-pain

http://www.posetech.com/

http://www.bigbarn.co.uk

http://www.vibramfivefingers.it/

http://robbwolf.com/

http://chriskresser.com/my-favorite-gourmet-paleo-recipe-sites

http://www.westonaprice.org/

http://barefootrunning.fas.harvard.edu

http://www.anatomyinmotion.co.uk

http://www.movenat.com

htto://www.paleohacks.com

http://biophile.co.za/topics

Lightning Source UK Ltd.
Milton Keynes UK
UKOW040600260412

191467UK00001B/13/P